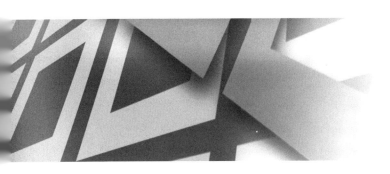

A Competency-Based Framework for Health Educators – 2006

The National Commission for Health Education
Credentialing, Inc.
Society for Public Health Education
American Association for Health Education

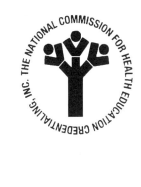

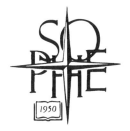

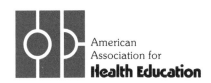

A Competency-Based Framework for Health Educators – 2006

For reprint permission or ordering information contact
The National Commission for Health Education Credentialing, Inc.
1541 Alta Drive, Suite 303 Whitehall PA 18052-5642
www.nchec.org   888-624-3248

Acknowledgments

This document is based on the results of the National Health Educator Competencies Update Project (CUP), which was conducted from 1998 through 2004. Historical information, as well as an interpretation of the CUP data, is included here to provide direction for the professional preparation and practice of health educators in a variety of settings.

As the joint copyright holders for this report, The CUP Technical Report, and the CUP data, the American Association for Health Education, the National Commission for Health Education Credentialing, Inc., and the Society for Public Health Education wish to acknowledge the following professionals for their contributions throughout the project. Their expertise, input, and dedication have achieved another significant milestone for the health education profession.

A Competency-Based Framework for Health Educators – 2006

Writers
Dr. Stephen Stewart (Committee Chair)
Dr. Donna Videto
Dr. Tom Butler
Dr. Susan Radius

Reviewers
Dr. Matthew Adeyanju
Ms. Elaine Auld
Dr. Michael Barnes
Dr. Marianne Frauenknecht
Dr. Gary Gilmore
Ms. Linda Lysoby
Dr. James McKenzie
Dr. Larry Olsen
Dr. Robert Simmons
Dr. Becky J. Smith
Dr. Alyson Taub
Dr. Lynn Woodhouse

Contributors
Dr. Carol Cox
Dr. Dixie Dennis
Ms. Andrea James
Dr. Beverly Mahoney

Copy-editor
Janis Foster

National Health Educator Competencies Update Project (CUP)

Steering Committee
Dr. Gary Gilmore, CUP Chair
Dr. Larry Olsen
Dr. Alyson Taub

Advisory Committee
Ms. Elaine Auld
Dr. David R. Black
Dr. Tom Butler
Dr. Ellen M. Capwell
Dr. Helen Welle Graf
Ms. Barbara Hager
Ms. Linda Lysoby
Dr. Beverly Mahoney
Dr. Mary Marks
Dr. Marion Micke
Dr. Kathleen Miner
Dr. Sheila M. Patterson
Dr. Susan Radius
Dr. Edmund Ricci
Dr. John Sciacca
Dr. Becky Smith
Dr. Margaret Smith
Dr. Carol Soha
Ms. Lori Stegmier
Dr. Stephen H. Stewart
Ms. Emily Tyler

CUP Data Analysis Group (2003-2004)
Dr. Randy Black
Dr. Dave Connell
Dr. Dan Coster
Dr. Gary Gilmore
Dr. Kathy Miner
Dr. Larry Olsen
Dr. Alyson Taub

Reviewers of the CUP Final Report
Dr. Collins Airhihenbuwa
Dr. John Allegrante
Dr. Randall Cottrell
Dr. Robert Gold
Dr. Bruce Simons-Morton
Dr. Mohammad Torabi

Table of Contents

Table of Contents (continued)

Introduction

Health education as a discipline has existed for approximately a century in the United States. Today, some 250 academic programs train health educators in the science and art of the profession (AAHE, 2005), and thousands of individuals—practitioners, academics, and researchers—view themselves as health educators. A solid foundation clearly exists for the preparation, evaluation, and credentialing of health educators (NCHEC, 1996).

Health education reached a new level of maturity with the publication of *A Framework for the Development of Competency-Based Curricula for Entry Level Health Educators* (NCHEC, 1985), which contained the responsibilities, competencies, and sub-competencies that became the standards for the profession. Another maturation milestone occurred 12 years later with the publication of *Standards for the Preparation of Graduate-Level Health Educators* (SOPHE & AAHE, 1997), which specified additional roles and competencies expected of the graduate health educator.

As in all professions, changing trends, changing environments, and changing populations necessitate alterations in how individuals perform their jobs. Thus, the National Health Educator Competencies Update Project (CUP) was launched in 1998 to identify what health educators do in practice, assess the degree to which the role definition of the entry-level health educator was up to date, and validate the graduate-level competencies. Thousands of health educators across the nation participated in this research, which was groundbreaking in its scope and technique. Thanks to the commitment of all who led and participated in the CUP research, a revised set of competencies for health educators at multiple levels of practice has emerged. This is the subject of this publication.

This document chronicles the evolution of professional standards for health education, the CUP process and research outcomes, and the application of an updated framework to health education students, faculty, practitioners, and other audiences. The National Commission for Health Education Credentialing, Inc. (NCHEC), the Society for Public Health Education (SOPHE), and the American Association for Health Education (AAHE) would like to express their sincere gratitude to the CUP Advisory Committee and especially the CUP Steering Committee — Dr. Gary D. Gilmore, Dr. Larry K. Olsen, and Dr. Alyson Taub — for their dedicated scholarship on the CUP study. Without their significant and enduring teamwork and careful stewardship, this new milestone in health education would not have been realized. ◆

Section I:
Historical Perspectives

Section I: Historical Perspectives

The National Health Educator Competencies Update Project (CUP) research was built on a previous body of work that helped to define health education practice and contributed to its "professionalization." This section presents relevant health education history in an effort to provide a context for the purpose of CUP, its methodologies, and the significance of its findings.

Health Education in the United States

The history of health education in the United States dates back to the late 19th century with the establishment of the first academic programs preparing school health educators (Allegrante et al., 2004). Interest in quality assurance and the development of standards for professional preparation of health educators emerged in the 1940s. Over the next several decades, professional associations produced guidelines for preparing health educators and accreditation efforts were introduced. Yet it was not until the 1970s that health education began evolving as a true profession in terms of a sociological perspective (Livingood & Auld, 2004). In addition to defining a body of literature, efforts were initiated to promulgate a health education code of ethics, a skill-based set of competencies, rigorous systems for quality assurance, and a health education credentialing system. Today some 250 academic programs in colleges and universities prepare health educators at the undergraduate and graduate levels leading to baccalaureate, master's, and doctoral degrees (AAHE, 2005). A profession-wide code of ethics has been endorsed and disseminated by the leading health education professional associations (CNHEO, 1999). Behavioral and social science research has provided a strong theoretical base for health education interventions, and professional associations have demonstrated that they can collaborate in defining and preparing health educators for contemporary workplace demands. According to NCHEC, more than 12,000 professionals have received the designation Certified Health Education Specialist (CHES) nationwide.

Competency-Based Approach

Long-standing questions about what health educators do in practice eventually led to the first Role Delineation Project in the 1970s. Prior investigations as well as the recent CUP research involved defining the health educator's role by delineating the competencies critical to success in that role. A competency-based approach helped to provide a framework of the skills and abilities needed to perform in a health educator position.

In 1985, the National Commission for Health Education Credentialing, Inc. (NCHEC) defined a competency as "an ability to apply a certain specified skill in dealing with some defined amount of meaningful subject matter" (p. 2). As such, competencies are a reflection of both content and process. Further noted was that competencies "describe broadly defined skills that a qualified ... generic health educator is expected to be able to demonstrate at least at minimum levels" (NCHEC, 1985, p. 2). Although the above definition was applied only to the entry-level health educator in previous research, it has relevance for all levels of practice in the CUP Model.

Background

Unlike most health professions, health education conducted a role delineation/verification/refinement process (Henderson & McIntosh, 1981; Cleary, 1997) that eventually resulted in verified competencies for health education practice (NCHEC, 1985). In

February 1978, the First Bethesda Conference assembled health educators from all practice settings to begin the process of defining and verifying the role of health educators. The stated purposes of the conference were 1) to analyze the commonalities and differences that existed in the preparation of health educators for different practice settings and 2) to determine the potential for developing acceptable guidelines for professional preparation that would include all practice settings (NCHEC, 1985). The conference's recommendation to establish the National Task Force on the Preparation and Practice of Health Educators was realized in March 1978, when the National Center for Health Education undertook the landmark Role Delineation Project (U.S. Department of Health, Education, and Welfare, 1978).

After considerable public discussion and background research, the role of the entry-level health education specialist was defined during the years 1978 to 1981. Responsibilities, functions, skills, and knowledge expected of the entry-level health educator were delineated. Thereafter, a national survey of practicing health educators was conducted to verify and refine the definition. The research showed that there was a "generic role" of all health educators; that is, there are commonalities in the roles of entry-level health educators regardless of whether they are employed in schools, communities, worksites, or other settings. This finding formed the basis for the credentialing process for heath educators.

Using the defined role, the National Task Force on the Preparation and Practice of Health Educators developed a curriculum framework during 1981 to 1985. This framework was based on contributions from academics and practitioners involved in two national conferences, several regional workshops, and many meetings of professional associations. The resulting document, *A Framework for the Development of Competency-Based Curricula for Entry-Level Health Educators* (NCHEC, 1985), provided professional preparation programs a frame of reference for developing their health education curricula. The CUP research continues to build on the work of both the Role Delineation Project and the National Task Force.

The Second Bethesda Conference in 1986 provided consensus that a certification process was appropriate to ensure that individuals delivering health education services possessed a minimal level of competency. Preliminary steps for developing a national certification system for health education specialists were initiated, culminating with the establishment of NCHEC in 1988.

Following a charter certification phase in 1989, during which practitioners could become certified through a review of documentation submitted by the individual (e.g., letters of support, academic records), the first national competency-based certification examination was offered by NCHEC in 1990. Thus, the competencies identified through this process formed the basis for a framework for professional preparation and a national examination, leading to credentialing the eligible individual as a CHES (NCHEC, 1996).

Efforts to determine graduate-level competencies were initiated in 1992 by the American Association for Health Education (AAHE) and the Society for Public Health Education (SOPHE), which commissioned the Joint Committee for the Development of Graduate-Level Preparation Standards. The committee sought the input of academics involved in graduate-level professional preparation through a national survey and at various annual meetings, as well as through its own continuing deliberations, to ascertain the advanced-level competencies practiced by health education specialists with advanced training and experience. It was projected that such competencies would build on the entry-level skills within the seven areas of responsibility that had been identified, as well as establish new areas of responsibility at the advanced level.

Following the publication of a final report (SOPHE & AAHE, 1997) and its acceptance by the boards of AAHE, NCHEC, and SOPHE, the Graduate Competencies Implementation Committee was formed. This committee addressed the manner in which the new advanced-level competencies would be disseminated to, and implemented by, the profession. The resulting document, *A Competency-Based Framework for Graduate-Level Health Educators,* was jointly published in 1999 by AAHE, NCHEC, and SOPHE. This publication contains a complete history of the development of the proposed advanced-level competencies.

During the mid- to late 1990s, professional organizations and individual health education specialists expressed a desire to re-verify the entry-level competencies to ensure that they reflected current health education research findings and practice; to further integrate, refine, and validate the advanced (graduate-level) competencies; and to add to the advanced competencies as appropriate. To this end, NCHEC initiated the National Health Educator Competencies Update Project (CUP) in 1998, with the participation of AAHE, SOPHE, and nine other national health education–related organizations. Preliminary discussions took place at the national convention of the American Alliance for Health, Physical Education, Recreation and Dance in Reno, Nevada, during April 1998. Once the CUP project was announced, two working groups were formed: 1) the Competencies Update Project Advisory Committee (CUPAC), which represented all of the major health education associations and provided guidance to the Competencies Update Project Steering Committee (CUPSC), and 2) the Competencies Update Data Analysis Group (CUPDAG), which provided statistical and methodological guidance in the CUP research.

During the remainder of 1998, efforts were devoted to planning the research and its support. The CUP organizing format was based on the previous work that defined areas of responsibility, competencies, and sub-competencies for professional practice (NCHEC, 1985). The challenge was in specifying the study questions, methodologies, and approaches to data analysis.

As the CUP investigation was beginning to take shape, SOPHE and AAHE convened an invitational meeting in 2000 of key health education leaders to explore various issues facing the profession in quality assurance, including a fragmented system of program approval processes and accreditation mechanisms (Allegrante et al, 2004). A critical recommendation from the meeting was that "a comprehensive, coordinated accreditation system for undergraduate and graduate health education should be put into place, which builds on the strengths of current mechanisms" (p. 672). Subsequently, a three-year task force developed principles and seven recommendations for strengthening both professional preparation and certification in health education. These recommendations have been widely disseminated to the profession and have relevance to the CUP research. In 2004, AAHE and SOPHE commissioned the National Transition Task Force on Accreditation in Health Education to help implement the recommendations. This group convened the "Third National Congress on Institutions Preparing Health Educators: Linking Program Assessment, Accountability and Improvement," February 23–25, 2006, in Dallas. In addition to reviewing recent accreditation developments, a central objective of the meeting was to disseminate the CUP Model and examine its implications for health education faculty, students, practitioners, employers, and other stakeholders. ◆

Section II:
The CUP Process and Outcomes

Section II: The CUP Process and Outcomes

Introduction

The National Health Educator Competencies Update Project (CUP) was a 6-year (1998-2004) multiphase national research study designed to re-verify the role of entry-level health educators and further define and verify the role of advanced-level health educators in the United States.[1] The project was guided by the CUP National Advisory Committee (CUPAC), which included representatives from 12 national professional groups with interests in health education.[2] The volunteer CUP Steering Committee (CUPSC) led the overall project, aided by a research consultant, a statistical consultant, and representatives of the CUPAC who provided specific expertise during the data analysis phase (CUP Data Analysis Group, or CUPDAG). Financial support for the research came from a variety of sources (i.e. professional associations, government, universities, and individuals) along with more than 10,000 hours of in-kind time. The CUP builds on previous work to define professional practice and contribute to the "professionalization" of health education (American Association for Health Education, National Commission for Health Education Credentialing, Inc. [NCHEC], & Society for Public Health Education, 1999; Cleary, 1995; Henderson & McIntosh, 1981; NCHEC, 1985, 1996).

CUP Methodology

The CUP project addressed the following four research questions:
1. What is the current generic role of the entry-level health education specialist compared with the role previously defined?
2. What are the generic areas of responsibility, competencies, and sub-competencies of advanced-level health education specialists?
3. Are there commonalities in the roles of entry-level and advanced-level health education specialists across practice settings?
4. Are there differences in the roles of entry-level and advanced-level health education specialists based on degrees held and years of work experience in health education?

The research questions were limited to what a health educator does in practice and did not investigate how well the health educator performed on the job. Questions about how well a practitioner performs given skills or the influence of one's preparation on attained skills were not addressed in this research. In addition, it should be noted that the study was designed to determine what health educators did at the time of the study, not what they thought they should be doing in the future.

The CUP research was conducted in several phases. During the planning phase (1998-1999), three fact-finding work groups composed of advisory committee members focused on levels of practice, proposed new competencies, and resource development. Following this work, a series of pre-pilot research activities were completed to develop a preliminary research instrument, to conduct a limited pilot of a draft research instrument, and to test alternative response modalities (e.g., postal mail vs. Web vs. e-mail).

A national pilot study was completed in four states (i.e. New York, Texas, Iowa, and Oregon) between June 2000 and September 2001 (Gilmore, Olsen, & Taub, 2001). States were randomly selected representing the four major census regions, including two states with a high concentration of health educators and two states with a low concentration of health educators. A random sample of 1,600 individuals in the four pilot states were sent a letter explaining the study, a list of the national advisory committee members, a background information form, and a postage-paid return envelope. The background information forms were designed to determine the eligibility of the potential respondents for the research. The respondents who self-identified as health educators, were currently working in health education, and were willing to participate received the CUP questionnaire by postal mail (with a business reply envelope). Potential participants were given the option of responding to the mailed questionnaire or completing the questionnaire on a Web site. Incentives for participation (e.g. book sets, professional memberships, and national convention registrations) were offered through a drawing. Numerous addresses were found to be inaccurate, out-of-date, or undeliverable. A telephone follow-up was conducted with a 10% random sample of non-respondents to determine reasons for not answering the questionnaire. The adjusted response rate was 76.1% (204 out of 268) of those who were eligible to complete the pilot survey. Findings from the pilot study emphasized the importance of accurate and up-to-date lists of health educators, use of home addresses whenever possible, the need to assure proportional representation from all work settings, and respondents' preference for a postal mail survey versus a Web-based approach to data collection.

During the major research phase from 2001 to 2004, questionnaires were sent to a representative sample of members of national professional organizations of health educators across all 50 states and the District of Columbia. In addition, in 16 randomly selected states (i.e., 2 states with high concentrations of health education practitioners and 2 with lower concentrations from each one of the four national regions), questionnaires were mailed to a random sample of individuals on lists solicited from state departments of education and public health, state affiliates of national health education organizations, allied health and medical care organizations, and other sources. Obtaining a nationally representative sample of health educators in the absence of a complete census of the population was extremely difficult. A two-step list acquisition process was developed for this research, which contributed to the representativeness of the sample by providing access to health educators in the major work settings, individuals who did not belong to national professional associations, and those working at local levels (Gilmore, Olsen, Taub, & Connell, 2004). Analysis of the data for the two samples revealed that there were no statistically significant differences in responses within comparable subgroups (e.g., comparing school health educators in each sample).

The 19-page questionnaire used in the study produced the largest national data set ever constructed from practicing health educators in the United States (more than 1.6 million data points). Questionnaires were completed by 4,030 health educators (70.6% adjusted response rate) from every state in the United States and the District of Columbia. Responding health educators were distributed across a wide array of work settings (e.g., community, school, college/university, health care, business/industry). The questionnaire was divided into three sections:

- Part A, Analysis of Activities, contained 180 items for which participants rated, on a 4-point scale, how frequently they performed each skill and how important each skill was to carrying out the responsibilities of their current position.

- Part B, Assessment of Responsibilities, contained items asking participants to approximate the percentage of time they spent carrying out each of 10 areas of responsibility and how important each of the 10 areas of responsibility was to their current job. Furthermore, participants were asked to rate, on a 3-point scale, under what conditions they were supervised as health educators or the conditions under which they supervised other health educators.
- Part C, Demographic Data, included items covering the participant's professional identity, present position, educational background, years of experience as a health educator, and type of organization where the respondent was presently employed.

The questionnaire was sent by postal mail, followed by postcard reminders. Incentives for participation, such as U.S. savings bonds, book sets, professional memberships, and national convention registrations, were offered through a drawing. A 10% non-respondent follow-up study was also completed (for details, see Gilmore, Olsen, & Taub, 2004).

Responses on each questionnaire were double-entered to ensure accuracy; all data were cleaned, verified, and reviewed. More than 95% of the respondents answered all items in the questionnaire, with less than 1% of the data missing.

Several important decisions were made before the analysis of the survey data could be completed. First, the frequency and importance ratings for each item were combined into a single "score." Second, following a review of the combined score data by the National Advisory Committee, 17 items were removed from further analysis because both frequency and importance ratings were extremely low (i.e., most respondents reported that the skill was infrequently performed and was not important for their job). Third, the CUP Data Analysis Group (CUPDAG) identified an advanced analysis process called Facets for appropriately converting ordinal data into interval data, enabling parametric analyses to be used. The Facets process estimates a linear measure, or logit, for each facet in the data. For the CUP research, respondents and items were the two facets. In keeping with item response theory (IRT), the Facets process addresses any instrument design and analysis flaw through the use of rating scale measurement models prior to using standard parametric analyses (Linacre, 1998, 1999, 2003; Rasch, 1990; Schulman, Trujillo, & Karney, 2001). The resulting "logit scores" were transformed to a scale ranging from 0 to 100 for ease of data assessment. More discussion of each of these decisions follows in the next section.

CUP Findings

Despite the difficulties in compiling the lists of health educators, the resulting sample of 4,030 respondents was considered to be the most representative sample of its kind. Almost 85% of the respondents reported working full-time in their current position. About 42% reported that 75% to 100% of their work time was as a health educator, and an additional 27% had duties as a health educator for 50% to 75% of their time. Thus, the majority of those included in the research reported health education as their primary role. More than 50% of the respondents reported that they had some administrative duties associated with their present position. Nearly 25% of the respondents ($n = 983$) who reported their years of experience in health education indicated they had less than 5 years of experience. Respondents with 5 or more years of experience reported, on average, 16.1 years of experience as a health educator and 8.3 years in their current position. A total of 3,993 respondents reported their current type of employer. As the results were reviewed, four major work settings (community, school/K-12, health care, university/professional preparation) emerged and were used in the data analyses. The business/industry work setting had too few respondents for any meaningful analysis. Also, there were no respondents in the university health service category.

For each work setting, except university/professional preparation, more than 60% of the respondents reported having master's degrees. For universities, more than half of the respondents reported having doctoral degrees. Furthermore, more than two thirds of all doctoral-level respondents (70.2%; 500 of 712) who completed the questionnaire reported being employed in the university/professional preparation work setting.

Responses to Part A of the survey provided 360 separate variables for analysis; that is, for each of the 180 items, a rating of both frequency and importance was provided. Correlations between frequency and importance ratings were very high, ranging from .62 to .83 across all 180 items (median .78, mean .79). The correlations between frequency and importance were between .62 and .69 for 9 of the items, 120 items correlated between .70 and .79, and the remaining 51 items correlated between .80 and .83. Each of these correlations was statistically significant beyond $p < .001$. Because the frequency and importance ratings consistently provided information that was similar and overlapping, the CUPDAG made a decision to combine those ratings for analysis by adding the two scores.

The CUPDAG members further agreed that the rating of importance should be given more weight than the rating of frequency in establishing a role description for health educators. This approach was supported by the CUPAC. The rationale was that a health educator might not be required to perform all skills in a particular job. The rating of importance of the skill to the current job was felt to be more pertinent. Therefore, the combined score for frequency and importance was computed as "Combined score = (frequency – 1) + importance."

The majority of items contained in the questionnaire were reported as being performed frequently as well as being skills that were important for the individual to carry out within his or her current job responsibilities. A small number of items, however, were rated as being neither performed frequently nor important to the individual's current job responsibilities. The CUPAC approved the following criterion to be applied when considering removal of an item from further consideration within the emerging model: Items where more than half the respondents from each of four primary work settings (community, school, health care, and university/professional preparation) did not have a combined score of 3 or higher would be dropped from further analysis.

The inclusion of four practice settings reflects the generic nature of the sub-competencies. The value of 3 was considered by the CUPAC to allow for reasonable inclusion of sub-competencies, without being too low or too high. In all, 17 sub-competencies were dropped from further analysis and consideration for inclusion in the emerging model. The rationale that guided the decision to keep or drop any given sub-competency was to favor inclusion rather than exclusion. This meant that for any given sub-competency to be dropped, respondents had to have indicated that the sub-competency was not important and that it was not performed frequently (e.g., the mean combined score for the item was less than 3). If the mean combined score for any given sub-competency was 3 or more for either of the experience groups, the item was retained.

Most test instruments, including the CUP questionnaire, record Likert-type responses on an ordinal scale, meaning that items are rank-ordered on a continuum. Nonparametric statistics, sometimes referred to as ranking statistics (e.g., Mann-Whitney U), are designed to be used with these data where the median is the central tendency of choice. When these scales are analyzed using standard parametric statistical methods appropriate for interval/ratio scales of measurement (e.g., ANOVA), it is assumed that the size of the interval between adjacent response options is the same for all response categories and all items. Thus, each response interval represents an equal amount of the underlying measured variable. However, those designing the item response options may not have intended that all response option intervals be considered equal. Furthermore, those responding to the sub-competencies also may have viewed the response option intervals as non-equal. In either circumstance, these perceptions may have produced distortions in the analyses and, consequently, led to misleading estimates and inferences.

IRT addresses the instrument design and analysis flaw presented above by first fitting rating scale measurement (RSM) models, for example, the RSM models developed by Rasch (1990), before using standard parametric analyses such as ANOVA, regression, and/or factor analysis (Schulman et al., 2001). Facets (Linacre, 1998, 1999, 2003) is one of a collection of programs created to implement Rasch models under IRT models. Specifically, Facets converts ordinal-scaled response data to interval/ratio scales by estimating a linear measure, or logit, for each facet in the data. In the case of CUP, there were two facets: respondents and items. The response scale was a 7-point Likert-type ordinal scale produced by combining the original importance and frequency item responses. For the CUP data, there was statistically significant separation among all seven ordered response categories, although, as expected, the separation was less in magnitude on the logit scale between central response categories than the separation between either extreme category and the nearest more-central response category. The Facets program provided an adjusted logit score for each response from each respondent. Across the entire data set, the mean score was 0.0, and the standard deviation was 1.0. The range of scores, again across all items and respondents, was from –2.28 to +2.13 (for a total range of 4.41). The CUPDAG then made a decision to simplify interpretation of the data by transforming each score so that the data set mean would be 50.0 and the scores would range from 0.0 to 100.0. This was accomplished through a simple linear transformation.

For a comparison of the areas of responsibility in the entry-level framework (1985), the graduate-level framework (1999), and the CUP Model (2006), see Table 1.

It should be noted that the sub-competencies aligned with each competency in the CUP Model include some of the statements from the two prior models (the original entry-level model and the graduate-level model), along with newly verified sub-competencies. Additionally, since the CUP Model differentiates three levels of practice (Entry, Advanced 1, and Advanced 2), each sub-competency was aligned with a specific level of practice within some competencies in the model. In some areas of responsibility, competencies do not have sub-competencies aligned with each level of practice.

To assess whether there were significant differences in self-reported frequency and importance ratings of the sub-competencies by years of experience as a health educator, a series of discriminate analyses were completed. The question addressed was: Is there a specific number of years of experience where health educators clearly begin to

Table 1. Comparison of Areas of Responsibility (1985-2006)*

Entry-Level Framework (1985)	Graduate-Level Framework (1999)	CUP Model (2006)
I. Assessing individual and community needs for health education	I. Assessing individual and community needs for health education	I. Assess individual and community needs for health education
II. Planning effective health education programs	II. Planning effective health education programs	II. Plan health education strategies, interventions, and programs
III. Implementing health education programs	III. Implementing health education programs	III. Implement health education strategies, interventions, and programs
IV. Evaluating effectiveness of health education programs	IV. Evaluating effectiveness of health education programs	IV. Conduct evaluation and research related to health education
V. Coordinating provision of health education services	V. Coordinating provision of health education services	V. Administer health education strategies, interventions, and programs
VI. Acting as a resource person in health education	VI. Acting as a resource person in health education	VI. Serve as a health education resource person
VII. Communicating health and health education needs, concerns, and resources	VII. Communicating health and health education needs, concerns, and resources	VII. Communicate and advocate for health and health education
	VIII. Applying appropriate research principles and techniques in health education	
	IX. Administering health education programs	
	X. Advancing the profession of health education	

NOTE: CUP = Competencies Update Project.

Table taken from "Overview of the National Health Educator Competencies Update Project, 1998-2004," by Gilmore, G.D., Olsen, L.K., Taub, A., & Connell, D. (2005). Health Education & Behavior, 32(6):725-737.

*In Gilmore. et al., (2005), this model was referred to as CUP Model (2004). No major changes have been made to the Areas of Responsibility. After editing and refinement of competencies and sub-competencies and associated documents, this information is made available for the first time in its entirety to the public with the printing of this document, "A Competency Based Framework for Health Educators-2006." Therefore this is now referred to as the CUP Model (2006).

attach more importance to, and practice with greater frequency, the various sub-competencies contained in the questionnaire? Based on these analyses, it was determined 5 years of experience was sufficiently robust to use as an appropriate demarcation between Entry-level and Advanced-level health educators.

In considering Entry versus Advanced levels of practice, it was decided that those indicating their highest degree was the associate degree ($n = 54$) would be dropped from further consideration in this study. The reason was that there are no recognized health education programs that offer the associate's degree as the entry into the practice of health education. Furthermore, those who possess only the associate's degree are not eligible to sit for the Certified Health Education Specialist examination. It was also decided that because there were only 41 individuals who possessed the doctoral degree who had less than 5 years of experience, these individuals would also be dropped from the Entry-level category and not be considered in subsequent analyses.

Within the advanced level of practice, clear differences in response patterns were evident between those who reported possessing a doctorate and other members of the advanced group. Overall, 70.2% of the respondents possessing a doctoral degree were located in academic settings. Among respondents with 5 or more years of experience, those with doctorates reported consistently higher logit scores for the 180 sub-competencies than those with either baccalaureate or master's degrees. As a result, the advanced level of practice was split into two segments. Those who had either a baccalaureate or master's degree and 5 or more years of experience were designated as Advanced 1. Those possessing a doctoral degree and 5 or more years of experience were designated as Advanced 2.

Over a period of several months, a series of emerging models of health educator roles were developed. The analytic process included both iterative statistical analyses and reviews incorporating professional judgment and reexamination of the data available from the survey of 4,030 respondents. Competency and sub-competency alignment was determined on the basis of preliminary and confirmatory factor analyses, confirmed by the review of the CUPAC. Sub-competency alignment with the levels of practice was determined by ANOVA analyses and preliminary and confirmatory factor analyses, confirmed by the review of the CUPAC. Detailed discussion of the analyses conducted for the CUP Model development and the placement of sub-competencies into areas of responsibility, sub-competencies into competencies, and sub-competencies into levels of practice is included in the CUP technical report (Gilmore, Olsen, & Taub, 2004). These processes were undertaken to use the best scientific methods and meet the needs of the profession.

Discussion

The CUP results were aligned into a hierarchical model, rather than the linear model that characterized the previous entry- and advanced-level models. All health educators reported performing the 163 sub-competencies identified through the research and that these sub-competencies were important in their current jobs. The placement of a sub-competency into a level of practice was based on the combined score of frequency and importance, considering years of experience and highest academic degree held. Those practicing at the Advanced 2 level would include those competencies and sub-competencies at both the Advanced 1 and Entry levels. Similarly, those practicing at the Advanced 1 level would include not only the Advanced 1 competencies and sub-competencies but also those competencies and sub-competencies at the Entry level. This hierarchical approach is presented in Table 2.

Table 2. CUP Model Hierarchical Approach

Level of Practice	Competencies/Sub-competencies
Entry (less than 5 years of experience; baccalaureate or master's degree)	Entry
Advanced 1 (5 or more years of experience; baccalaureate or master's degree)	Entry + Advanced 1
Advanced 2 (doctorate and 5 or more years of experience)	Entry + Advanced 1 + Advanced 2

NOTE: CUP = Competencies Update Project.

Table taken from "Overview of the National Health Educator Competencies Update Project, 1998-2004," by Gilmore, G.D., Olsen, L.K., Taub, A., & Connell, D. (2005). Health Education & Behavior, 32(6):725-737.

Entry Level

In answering research question 1, the multiplicity of analyses, coupled with professional judgment, indicated that many of the entry-level sub-competencies initially identified in the Role Delineation Project (1980-1981) were still valid. However, there were some sub-competencies that were reported as being more important and more frequently performed by Advanced 1 or Advanced 2 level health educators. The validated, competency-based hierarchical model, referred to as the CUP Model, shows the three levels of practice and the sub-competencies, by competency and area of responsibility. Although the role of the Entry-level health educator appears to be similar to the role previously defined, one should note in the CUP Model that there are some competencies that contain no sub-competencies or only one or two sub-competencies. This suggests that the profession is continuing to emerge. Additional sub-competencies will most likely evolve in the future.

Of the 79 entry-level sub-competencies from the original entry-level model, 3 were deleted in the CUP research. With the new sub-competencies added, the CUP Model contains 82 sub-competencies at the Entry level.

Advanced Levels

In response to research question 2, analysis of the data revealed that certain sub-competencies were performed more frequently and considered more important to the job and thus were placed in the Advanced 1 or Advanced 2 levels of practice. The analysis not only differentiates entry from advanced levels of practice but also suggests that there are two advanced levels of practice. The CUP Model shows that at the advanced levels, some competencies contain none or one or two sub-competencies. These gaps suggest that additional sub-competencies might be added through future research.

Health educators at the Advanced 1 level should be able to perform all of the 82 Entry-level sub-competencies, along with the 48 Advanced 1 sub-competencies. Advanced 2 health educators should be able to perform all 163 sub-competencies, representing all three levels of practice.

Of the 81 advanced sub-competencies from the graduate-level framework, 12 were deleted through the CUP research process. With the new sub-competencies from the CUP research, there are 48 Advanced 1 sub-competencies and 33 Advanced 2 sub-competencies.

Generic Role

Research question 3 dealt with whether there were commonalities in the roles of entry- and advanced-level health educators across practice settings. This question deals with the generic nature of the sub-competencies, that is, those sub-competencies performed frequently and reported to be important in the current job by health educators in all work settings. In the data analysis, 50% or more of the respondents across the four work settings had to have a combined frequency and importance mean score of 3 or more for an item to be considered generic. All 163 sub-competencies contained in the CUP Model are generic, as demonstrated by the analytic information contained in the CUP technical report (Gilmore, Olsen, & Taub, 2004).

Levels of Practice

Research question 4 dealt with whether there were differences in the roles of entry- and advanced-level health education specialists based on degrees held and years of work experience in health education. The 163 sub-competencies represent what health educators at various levels of professional preparation and various levels of experience reported they do, and the relative importance of each of the sub-competencies to their current position as a health educator. The data analysis showed that those who possess the doctoral degree, for the most part, also reported more years of experience as a health educator than those with either a baccalaureate or master's degree.

For data analysis, the questionnaire item that was used as the independent variable was as follows: "How long have you worked as a health educator?" The research was designed to determine how long the individual had been in the field and to determine what health educators were doing now, not what they did many years previously. The data show that there are some differences in terms of years of experience as a health educator. However, in terms of degree held, those with the doctoral degree were clearly a separate group. It should be stressed again that the majority of those who held the doctoral degree were employed in university settings, and the majority of those individuals reported having 5 or more years of experience as a health educator. In addition, based on self-report of frequency of performance and importance of a given sub-competency in one's current position, there were no significant differences between the responses of health educators who possessed the baccalaureate or the master's degree, based on years of experience. It is important to note that although there were no significant differences by degree level (other than the doctorate), the relative competence or skill with which each of the sub-competencies is performed by those possessing these two degrees was not examined in the present research.

In the CUP Model, three levels of practice were identified through the research. This model statistically shows that there are differences in the roles of Entry- and Advanced-level health educators based on the degrees held and the years of experience of the individual. This difference is most evident when the individual reported having 5 or more years of experience and was particularly clear for individuals prepared at the doctoral level.

Limitations

The limitations inherent in the CUP research are the following:

- There is no complete list of all health educators in the United States from which to draw a nationally representative sample. Consequently, methods were used to identify currently practicing health educators in every state and the District of Columbia so that a random sample could be selected. The resulting sample was considered to be the most representative sample of its kind available at the time of the research.
- Research participants self-identified as health educators. The majority of those included in the research reported health education as their primary role.
- The results are based on responses from health educators willing to participate in the study and complete the 19-page questionnaire. Despite the use of membership lists from business/industry and university health service work settings and extensive follow-up procedures, there were too few respondents from the business/industry work setting for any meaningful analysis and no respondents in the university health service category.

Source: This section was adapted from "Overview of the National Health Educator Competencies Update Project, 1998-2004," by G.D. Gilmore, L.K. Olsen, A. Taub, and D. Connell, 2005, *Health Education & Behavior*, 2005, 32(6):725-737.

Notes

1. The Competencies Update Project (CUP) research results are jointly owned by the American Association for Health Education, the National Commission for Health Education Credentialing, Inc. and the Society for Public Health Education.

2. The CUP National Advisory Committee (CUPAC) included representatives from the following organizations: American Association for Health Education (AAHE); American Public Health Association, Public Health Education & Health Promotion Section (APHA-PHEHP); American Public Health Association, School Health Education & Services Section (APHA-SHES); American School Health Association (ASHA); Association of Schools of Public Health (ASPH); Association of State & Territorial Directors of Health Promotion & Public Health Education (currently called Directors of Health Promotion and Education); Council on Education for Public Health (CEPH); Coalition of National Health Education Organizations (CNHEO); Eta Sigma Gamma (ESG); National Commission for Health Education Credentialing, Inc. (NCHEC); Society for Public Health Education, Inc. (SOPHE); Society of State Directors of Health, Physical Education, and Recreation. ◆

Section III:
The CUP Model

Section III: The CUP Model

The CUP Model provides a common set of competencies for the development, assessment, and improvement of professional preparation, credentialing procedures, and professional development for health educators. As in earlier versions, the CUP competencies and sub-competencies are considered generic and independent of the setting in which the health educator works. This consideration does not imply that different sites of practice do not have unique requirements and expectations for their health education specialists.

These differences can and should be incorporated into the scope and sequence of the entire curriculum of professional preparation programs. For example, those planning to work in a community health agency might need more preparation in public health policy-making, while those preparing for high school teaching may need added emphasis on teaching techniques.

Unlike earlier versions, however, the CUP Model provides distinct sets of competencies and sub-competencies for the three levels of practice (i.e., Entry, Advanced 1, and Advanced 2). While the CUP findings differentiate the levels based on experience, it is important to note that the Coalition of National Health Education Organizations endorsed recommendations that direct baccalaureate programs in health education to prepare their graduates to perform the entry level competencies and sub-competencies. Also graduate level programs should prepare their graduates to perform the Advanced 1 and Advanced 2 competencies and sub-competencies as appropriate to the degree level. In addition, graduate level programs also should address all of the entry-level competencies and sub-competencies in the new hierarchical model. The specific recommendations are found in Section IV of this publication.

The competencies and sub-competencies align with seven areas of responsibility. An area of responsibility is defined as "one of the major categories of performance expectations of a proficient health education practitioner. The areas of responsibility define the scope of practice" (SOPHE & AAHE, 1997).

The areas of responsibility outlined in the CUP Model are:

I. Assess Individual and Community Needs for Health Education

II. Plan Health Education Strategies, Interventions, and Programs

III. Implement Health Education Strategies, Interventions, and Programs

IV. Conduct Evaluation and Research Related to Health Education

V. Administer Health Education Strategies, Interventions, and Programs

VI. Serve as a Health Education Resource Person

VII. Communicate and Advocate for Health and Health Education

National Health Educator Competencies Update Project (CUP): CUP Competency-Based Hierarchical Model[1]

Area I: Assess Individual and Community Needs for Health Education

	Entry (Baccalaureate/master's, less than 5 years' experience)	**Advanced 1** (Baccalaureate/master's, 5 years' experience or more)	**Advanced 2** (Doctorate and 5 years' experience or more)
Competency A: Access existing health-related data	1. Identify diverse health-related databases 2. Use computerized sources of health-related information 3. Determine the compatibility of data from different data sources 4. Select valid sources of information about health needs and interests	. . .	1. Critique sources of health information
Competency B: Collect health-related data	1. Use appropriate data-gathering instruments 2. Apply survey techniques to acquire health data 3. Conduct health-related needs assessments 4. Implement appropriate measures to assess capacity for improving health status	. . .	. . .
Competency C: Distinguish between behaviors that foster or hinder well-being	1. Identify diverse factors that influence health behaviors 2. Identify behaviors that tend to promote or compromise health	1. Explain the role of experiences in shaping patterns of health behavior	. . .
Competency D: Determine factors that influence learning	. . .	1. Assess learning literacy 2. Assess learning styles	1. Assess the learning environment
Competency E: Identify factors that foster or hinder the process of health education	1. Determine the extent of available health education services 2. Identify gaps and overlaps in the provision of collaborative health services	1. Assess the environmental and political climate (e.g., organizational, community, state, and national) regarding conditions that advance or inhibit program goals	1. Investigate social forces causing opposing viewpoints regarding health education needs and concerns
Competency F: Infer needs for health education from obtained data	1. Analyze needs assessment data	1. Determine priorities for health education	1. Predict future health education needs based upon societal changes

[1] In the CUP model, derived from extensive national research, each level of practice builds on the previous level(s). Competencies in some areas of responsibility do not have sub-competencies aligned with each level of practice. Future research may yield additional sub-competencies. There are two duplicate subcompetencies in Area IV because two identical items appeared on the questionnaire used in the research. See the CUP technical report (Gilmore, Olsen, & Taub, 2004) for more in-depth discussion of model development. This model is copyrighted by the American Association for Health Education, the National Commission for Health Education Credentialing, and the Society for Public Health Education.

Area of Responsibility I: Assess Individual and Community Needs for Health Education

The Role. The primary purpose of a needs assessment is to gather information to determine what health education activities are appropriate in a given setting. Needs may be basic—that is, essential to the comfort and well-being of every human being (food, water, warmth, oxygen, etc.)—or indicators of a gap between conditions as they are and as they ought to be. Although the term "problem" is frequently used interchangeably with "need" in health education, strictly speaking they are different. A health problem is defined as a potential or real threat to physical or emotional well-being, amelioration or removal of which is a need.

Needs assessment is the systematic, planned collection of information about the health knowledge, perceptions, attitudes, motivation, and practices of individuals or groups and the quality of the socioeconomic environment in which they live. Assessing needs logically should precede program planning. This process provides data that determine whether a health education program is justified, and if so what its nature and emphasis ought to be.

To successfully conduct a needs assessment, it is necessary to be able to identify health-related databases and computerized and valid sources of data. It is also necessary to be able to gather data with appropriate instruments, apply survey techniques, and identify behaviors that influence health. Determining the extent of existing services and gaps in the provision of services is critical, along with the need to be able to analyze data and determine priorities for health education.

Settings.

Community Setting. The health educator in the community draws on many sources of current data, such as health planning agencies, public health departments, census reports, and interviews obtained from community leaders as well as from members of the priority population. These data provide information about perceived health needs. If specific behaviors or health practices are causally linked to the incidence of major health problems, then a health education program may be planned to motivate and facilitate voluntary, desirable changes in those behaviors.

School (K-12) Setting. In the school setting, local, state, and national data are used to determine the scope and sequence of curricula and to identify weaknesses in developing a coordinated school health program. National-level and state-level data should be considered and utilized, but local data are essential to good curriculum planning. Information about health knowledge, attitudes, skills and practices can be gathered directly from students and utilized to improve health instruction, school policies, and the school environment. Information gathered from parents, administrators, and school health personnel by a "Healthy School Team," consisting of representatives from each of the eight components of the Coordinated School Health Program, will assist in identifying potential gaps in creating a healthy school community.

Health Care Setting. In the health care setting, complaints by health professionals about a growing number of emergency room visits, for example, might lead the health educator to survey records to pinpoint the extent to which the problem is general or limited to patients with particular kinds of emergencies or with situational needs (e.g., patients without adequate health insurance or with limited access to primary care physicians). An assessment of the reasons for this trend would help to determine what services or policies could help to improve the situation.

Business/Industry Setting. In the workplace, a health educator might work with medical professionals to analyze employee records that can be used to identify health needs of the workers; for example, data about health insurance claims, absenteeism and its causes, types of accidents and severity of injuries, and compensation claims. In addition, a health educator in this setting should survey employees to discover their felt needs and interests. Analysis of these data would indicate priority needs for health promotion programs.

College/University Setting. In the college or university setting, health educators are often involved in assessing student performance in meeting state and national standards in order to maintain accreditation. Tracking students' progress in meeting the standards, assessing the learning environment, and linking the two are important for revising the curriculum and meeting accreditation requirements.

University Health Services Setting. The health educator who practices in student health services works side by side with clinical practitioners. The health educator assesses the health needs of students, staff, and faculty through the use of focus groups, surveys, and interviews. In the assessment process, it is important to develop avenues for obtaining information on perceptions, attitudes, practices, and felt needs in addition to health problems and practices

Area II: Plan Health Education Strategies, Interventions, and Programs

	Entry (Baccalaureate/master's, less than 5 years' experience)	Advanced 1 (Baccalaureate/master's, 5 years' experience or more)	Advanced 2 (Doctorate and 5 years' experience or more)
Competency A: Involve people and organizations in program planning	1. Identify populations for health education programs 2. Elicit input from those who will affect, or be affected by, the program 3. Obtain commitments from individuals who will be involved in the program 4. Develop plans for promoting collaborative efforts among health agencies and organizations with mutual interests	1. Involve participants in planning health education programs	...
Competency B: Incorporate data analysis and principles of community organization	1. Use research results when planning programs 2. Apply principles of community organization when planning programs 3. Suggest approaches for integrating health education within existing health programs 4. Communicate need for the program to those who will be involved	1. Incorporate results of needs assessment into the planning process	...
Competency C: Formulate appropriate and measurable program objectives	1. Design developmentally appropriate interventions	1. Establish criteria for health education program objectives 2. Develop program objectives based upon identified needs 3. Appraise appropriateness of resources and materials relative to given objectives 4. Revise program objectives as necessitated by changing needs	1. Develop subordinate measurable objectives as needed for instruction 2. Evaluate the efficacy of various methods to achieve objectives
Competency D: Develop a logical scope and sequence plan for health education practice	1. Determine the range of health information necessary for a given program of instruction 2. Select references relevant to health education issues or programs	1. Organize the subject areas comprising the scope of a program in logical sequence 2. Analyze the process for integrating health education into other programs	1. Incorporate theory-based foundations in planning health education programs

Area II: Plan Health Education Strategies, Interventions, and Programs (contunued)

	Entry (Baccalaureate/master's, less than 5 years' experience)	Advanced 1 (Baccalaureate/master's, 5 years' experience or more)	Advanced 2 (Doctorate and 5 years' experience or more)
Competency E: **Design strategies, interventions, and programs consistent with specified objectives**	...	1. Plan a sequence of learning opportunities that reinforce mastery of preceding objectives 2. Select strategies best suited to achieve objectives in a given setting	1. Formulate a variety of educational methods 2. Match proposed learning activities with stated program objectives 3. Select appropriate theory-based strategies in health program planning
Competency F: **Select appropriate strategies to meet objectives**	1. Analyze technologies, methods, and media for their acceptability to diverse groups 2. Match health education services to proposed program activities	1. Plan training and instructional programs for diverse populations 2. Incorporate communication strategies into program planning	1. Select educational materials consistent with accepted theory
Competency G: **Assess factors that affect implementation**	1. Determine the availability of information and resources needed to implement health education programs for a given audience 2. Identify barriers to the implementation of health education programs	1. Analyze factors (e.g., learner characteristics, legal aspects, feasibility) that influence choices among implementation methods 2. Select implementation strategies based upon research results	...

SECTION: III

Area of Responsibility II: Plan Health Education Strategies, Interventions, and Programs

The Role. Program planning begins with the assessment of existing health needs, problems, and concerns. The extent to which these are directly linked to health behaviors determines the specific changes in behaviors for which the program planning process is set in motion. Relevant people are identified and involved in the project, objectives are established, educational methods selected and resources located. It is within this process that planning for program evaluation is begun as well.

Settings.

Community Setting. In a community setting in which a needs assessment has identified a particular and significant health problem, the health educator convenes representatives of relevant groups to identify populations in need of health education; seeks input and promotes involvement from those who will affect and be affected by the program; uses research and the results of the needs assessment and applies principles of community organization to develop ways of integrating health education within existing health programs; formulates objectives and designs interventions appropriate to the population; and identifies and assesses community resources and barriers affecting implementation of the program. The selection of program activities and interventions depends on the characteristics of the priority population, their constraints and concerns, and the fit between program schedules and other obligations of the participants.

School (K-12) Setting. The decision to provide health education in schools is usually made by administrators or mandated by law. The school health educator organizes an advisory committee (consisting of teachers, administrators, members of the community, representatives from voluntary agencies, parents, youth group leaders, clergy, and students) to select or develop health education curricula and materials. These decisions should be based on research results and best practices and should consider available resources and barriers to implementation, such as time and space. Objectives should be based on the needs of school-aged children and young adults. Curricula should follow a logical scope and sequence.

Health Care Setting. The health educator in a health care setting works with nurses, physicians, nutritionists, physical therapists, and other health care professionals to plan patient and community education programs. The team develops education programs for patients and their families to promote compliance with medical directions and enhance understanding of medical procedures and conditions. The role of the health educator in this setting is to assist the team in establishing behavioral objectives, identifying roles of staff in providing education, selecting teaching methods and strategies, evaluating results, documenting the education effort, designing promotion activities, and training interdisciplinary staff to conduct the program, as appropriate.

Business/Industry Setting. In the workplace, the health educator analyzes data from numerous sources (including insurance records, safety records, workers' compensation claims, and employee self-report questionnaires) to provide a basis for a presentation to management outlining the benefits and costs of a health education program. After gaining administrative support, the health educator convenes an employee committee with representatives from all levels of the organization to make recommendations concerning program priorities, objectives, scheduling, publicity, incentives, and fees. The health educator leads the team in developing data- and theory-based interventions and strategies to meet the needs of employees.

College/University Setting. The health educator in a higher education setting analyzes research results, current professional competencies, accreditation standards, and certification requirements and uses the results to design professional preparation programs that will encourage the development of essential competencies in candidates regardless of future practice setting.

University Health Services Setting. The health educator who practices in student health services works side by side with clinical practitioners. The health educator uses the needs assessment to develop program and behavioral objectives and to design interventions that reduce health risks and improve health. The health educator works with clinical practitioners and others to integrate health education into other programs, including treatment regimens and campus-wide activities. He or she also evaluates the efficacy of educational methods to achieve objectives.

Area III: Implement Health Education Strategies, Interventions, and Programs

	Entry (Baccalaureate/master's, less than 5 years' experience)	**Advanced 1** (Baccalaureate/master's, 5 years' experience or more)	**Advanced 2** (Doctorate and 5 years' experience or more)
Competency A: Initiate a plan of action	1. Use community organization principles to facilitate change conducive to health 2. Pretest learners to determine baseline data relative to proposed program objectives 3. Deliver educational programs to diverse populations 4. Facilitate groups	1. Apply individual or group process methods as appropriate to given learning situations	. . .
Competency B: Demonstrate a variety of skills in delivering strategies, interventions, and programs	1. Use instructional technology effectively 2. Apply implementation strategies	1. Select methods that best facilitate achievement of program objectives 2. Apply technologies that will contribute to program objectives	1. Use a variety of educational methods
Competency C: Use a variety of methods to implement strategies, interventions, and programs	1. Use the Code of Ethics in professional practice 2. Apply theoretical and conceptual models from health education and related disciplines to improve program delivery 3. Demonstrate skills needed to develop capacity for improving health status 4. Incorporate demographically and culturally sensitive techniques when promoting programs 5. Implement intervention strategies to facilitate health-related change	1. Employ appropriate strategies when dealing with controversial health issues	. . .
Competency D: Conduct training programs	. . .	1. Demonstrate a wide range of strategies for conducting training programs	1. Use instructional resources that meet a variety of training needs

Area of Responsibility III: Implement Health Education Strategies, Interventions, and Programs

The Role. Health educators educate and motivate people in their pursuit of healthful behaviors. Regardless of the setting in which they work, health educators must be able to conduct programs as planned, infer objectives suitable to the program, select media and methods appropriate to the intended audience, and make revisions to programs and objectives consistent with results from having monitored their programs in action.

Settings.

Community Setting. Health educators working in the community face the challenge of motivating a diverse population to pursue healthful behaviors. Program objectives, the means of communicating those objectives, and the means of motivating changes in behavior should all take into account the needs, interests, and education of the target group. A health educator attempting to improve families' dietary choices, for example, might work with a local grocery chain to provide educational materials, hold a cooking demonstration at a community center, start a community vegetable garden or farmer's market, or work with schools to change vending machine policies.

School (K-12) Setting. In the school setting, health educators work to increase students' knowledge and promote positive attitudes and behaviors with respect to health. Provided with a curriculum by school administration, the school-based health educator infers objectives appropriate to students' learning potential and abilities and decides on appropriate teaching techniques. Lesson plans are informed by the health educator's awareness of the students' learning needs, degree of parental support, and related factors. Students' learning is monitored to facilitate revisions in the curriculum and instruction methods. The health educator also works with administrative staff and faculty and parent groups to encourage school policies that support healthy behaviors.

Health Care Setting. Health educators employed in health care settings function as independent participants as well as liaisons between patients and providers. A health educator in this setting might conduct a program to support patients' weight loss efforts. He or she might offer classes, supported by presentations from the health care providers and making use of educational materials consistent with the patients' needs. The health educator would monitor outcomes and patients' and providers' reactions, making changes to the program and objectives as warranted.

Business/Industry Setting. In the workplace, health educators work with employers to offer educational programs that respond to employees' health needs (e.g., programs to improve diet) in a manner conducive to employee participation. Employees might be offered healthful food choices in the company cafeteria, exercise classes, stress reduction counseling, and smoking cessation therapy, all supplemented by educational materials.

College/University Setting. A health educator working in a higher education setting might conduct an introductory-level health class in which he or she guides each student through a personal change project tailored to the student's interests, preparedness for the course, and learning style. Objectives of the project would be determined and modified, as needed, to fit the needs of both the student and the class. PowerPoint presentations, films, and role-playing are among the instructional methods that might be used. Student feedback and instructor observations can be used to refine future programs to more effectively achieve goals within the course's curriculum.

University Health Services Setting. In conjunction with health care providers, health educators in a university health services setting work with the entire university community. Programs are constructed in response to established needs of faculty, staff, and students. For example, with the support of appropriate university personnel, the health educator might work with residence officials to offer educational sessions in student dormitories on the topic of contraception. Program availability would match student needs and be supported by media intended to appeal to the college student. Incentives could be offered to encourage attendance. The health educator would monitor students' interest and attendance and request feedback from students and instructors to improve future programs.

Area IV: Conduct Evaluation and Research Related to Health Education

	Entry (Baccalaureate/master's, less than 5 years' experience)	Advanced 1 (Baccalaureate/master's, 5 years' experience or more)	Advanced 2 (Doctorate and 5 years' experience or more)
Competency A: **Develop plans for evaluation and research**	1. Synthesize information presented in the literature 2. Evaluate research designs, methods, and findings presented in the literature	1. Develop an inventory of existing valid and reliable tests and survey instruments	1. Assess the merits and limitations of qualitative and quantitative methods
Competency B: **Review research and evaluation procedures**	1. Evaluate data-gathering instruments and processes 2. Develop methods to evaluate factors that influence shifts in health status	1. Identify standards of performance to be applied as criteria of effectiveness 2. Identify methods to evaluate factors that influence shifts in health status 3. Select appropriate methods for evaluating program effectiveness	1. Establish a realistic scope of evaluation efforts 2. Select appropriate qualitative and/or quantitative evaluation design
Competency C: **Design data collection instruments**	1. Develop valid and reliable evaluation instruments 2. Develop appropriate data-gathering instruments	. . .	. . .
Competency D: **Carry out evaluation and research plans**	1. Use appropriate research methods and designs in health education practice 2. Use data collection methods appropriate for measuring stated objectives 3. Implement appropriate qualitative and quantitative evaluation techniques 4. Implement methods to evaluate factors that influence shifts in health status	1. Assess the relevance of existing program objectives to current needs	1. Apply appropriate evaluation technology 2. Analyze evaluation data
Competency E: **Interpret results from evaluation and research**	1. Analyze evaluation data 2. Analyze research data 3. Compare evaluation results to other findings 4. Report effectiveness of programs in achieving proposed objectives	1. Compare program activities with the stated program objectives 2. Develop recommendations based upon evaluation results	1. Determine the achievement of objectives by applying criteria to evaluation results 2. Communicate evaluation results using easily understood terms
Competency F: **Infer implications from findings for future health-related activities**	. . .	1. Suggest strategies for implementing recommendations that result from evaluation 2. Apply evaluation findings to refine and maintain programs	1. Propose possible explanations for evaluation findings

Area of Responsibility IV: Conduct Evaluation and Research Related To Health Education

The Role. Health educators at all levels are expected to be able to conduct a thorough review of the literature and to apply research findings from both basic and evaluative research. Health educators also may be expected to conduct evaluations of projects and programs. As the health educator progresses within the profession, the level of skill in conducting research and evaluation becomes more advanced. Health educators may be expected to write applications for funding, including research proposals. The ability to evaluate a program's effectiveness is essential to maintaining its funding in an increasingly competitive work environment. The ability to aggregate data from one or more programs for the purpose of establishing baselines and making comparisons is also important. Advanced-level health educators should be able to draw on various measures to establish the economic impacts of health education and health promotion programs; should be able to help identify other professionals needed for collaborative approaches; and should be able to provide information to governments, employers, and program funding sources. They should be able to translate research findings into lay language, making health communications more credible.

Settings.

Community Setting. The health educator may use epidemiological principles to explain disease outbreaks or define high-risk neighborhoods within communities that require special program emphasis. Evaluations may provide necessary information to support programs when reviewed by local or state governments. Research funding obtained by submitting competitive proposals not only may bring in revenue but may further encourage collaborative projects. The discussion of any topic important to the community, such as unintentional injuries, an outbreak of measles or food poisoning, or sexually transmitted diseases, requires mastery of research principles and language.

School (K-12) Setting. Health educators practicing in the school setting may be called upon to assist in the documentation of student health behaviors, knowledge, and attitudes. Data gained from a review of the literature and from qualitative and quantitative research are provided by health educators to school boards and parents to help them understand students' needs and interests. Careful use of research approaches also can help dispel intolerance relating to attitudes and behaviors maintained by a small but vocal population. Evaluation of curriculum goals, objectives, and learning activities is critical to identifying, selecting, and implementing effective curricula. Qualitative as well as quantitative research methods are increasingly being emphasized in school settings.

Health Care Setting. A health educator practicing in a health care setting must be able to understand and interpret research findings for patients and their families as well as participate as a member of a research team that investigates behavioral components of adherence to clinical regimens. As medical technologies and treatments are advanced through the conduct of clinical trials, evaluative research becomes increasingly important in addressing chronic disease conditions and the reduction of health risk behaviors.

Business/Industry Setting. Adults spend the majority of their time in the workplace. Health educators in this setting need both qualitative and quantitative research skills to demonstrate the efficacy of worksite health promotion programs and the contributions of such programs to productivity and organizational goals. Health educators also may be asked to assist in monitoring the work environment for safety compliance and injury reduction. Additionally, using evaluative research, health educators may be able to help determine both quality and cost-effectiveness of competing health plans to benefit both employers and employees.

College/University Setting. Health educators are expected to engage in scholarly endeavors that include research, grant writing, and dissemination of research findings. In addition to instructional and administrative responsibilities, university health educators frequently collaborate with others within and outside their respective institutions. These efforts contribute to the scientific body of knowledge on health behavior, disease prevention, and risk reduction strategies and to the discipline of health education.

University Health Services Setting. Health educators working in the university health services setting face many of the same issues as those in the business/Industry and the health care settings. These health educators need skills in all facets of research, qualitative and quantitative. Skill in evaluative research is necessary to determine the efficacy and cost-effectiveness of programs targeted to faculty, staff, and students.

Area V: Administer Health Education Strategies, Interventions, and Programs

	Entry (Baccalaureate/master's, less than 5 years' experience)	Advanced 1 (Baccalaureate/master's, 5 years' experience or more)	Advanced 2 (Doctorate and 5 years' experience or more)
Competency A: Exercise organizational leadership	1. Conduct strategic planning 2. Analyze the organization's culture in relationship to program goals 3. Promote cooperation and feedback among personnel related to the program	1. Develop strategies to reinforce or change organizational culture to achieve program goals 2. Ensure that program activities comply with existing laws and regulations 3. Develop budgets to support program requirements	1. Facilitate administration of the evaluation plan
Competency B: Secure fiscal resources	…	1. Manage program budgets	1. Prepare proposals to obtain fiscal resources
Competency C: Manage human resources	1. Develop volunteer opportunities	1. Demonstrate leadership in managing human resources 2. Apply human resource policies consistent with relevant laws and regulations 3. Identify qualifications of personnel needed for programs 4. Facilitate staff development 5. Apply appropriate methods of conflict reduction	…
Competency D: Obtain acceptance and support for programs	…	1. Use concepts and theories of public relations and communications to obtain program support 2. Facilitate cooperation among personnel responsible for health education programs	1. Provide support for individuals who deliver professional development courses

Area of Responsibility V: Administer Health Education Strategies, Interventions, and Programs

The Role. While some small administrative functions may fall to the entry-level health educator, administration is generally a function of the more experienced individual. Experienced health educators often become program managers or supervisors of other health educators or teams of allied health professionals. Good management and supervisory skills require training in a variety of organizational, psychological, and business environments. Good management incorporates effective "people skills" and knowledge of budgeting, task assignments, and performance evaluation. Supervisors answer to higher-level management as well as to staff. These individuals require effective communication skills, organizational knowledge, and objectivity. Because of their broad training and their understanding of individuals and communities, health educators can be effective managers who consider staff in the larger context of their institution or environment.

Settings.

Community Setting. Health educators in a community setting may be responsible for managing a program of several professional and paraprofessional health educators and outreach workers who provide programs and explain health agency initiatives. More experienced health educators may advance beyond specific health education/promotion programs and find themselves directing staff in other divisions of their local public health departments, such as mental health services, environmental health services, or health planning efforts.

School (K-12) Setting. In addition to managing classrooms of students, advanced-level health educators in the school setting now find themselves taking on greater responsibility in identifying and securing resources to support comprehensive school health programs. Serving as curriculum coordinators or project directors, health educators may manage curricular and budgetary issues for the school health program and may work with community agencies in providing selected content areas for students and staff. A frequent responsibility of the practicing health educator is the supervision of pre-service interns (student teachers). As curriculum specialists or program heads, health educators serve as team leaders to promote comprehensive health education in their school, throughout the school district, and at the state level.

Health Care Setting. Advanced health educators may be the managers of staff development programs in major medical complexes, nursing homes, or transitional facilities. The ability to communicate with a variety of medical professionals, aides, volunteers, clients, and family or community members is very important in this setting. Planning programs that contribute to institutional maintenance of accreditation and compliance with government regulations also may be the task of the health educator, who may supervise institutional service learning activities that augment staff efforts.

Business/Industry Setting. In this setting, a health educator at the advanced level may be part of a team as a coordinator for an employee assistance programs or director of a multi-staff health promotion effort. As an employee, a health educator may also supervise directly employed staff or contracted staff in health promotion programs (e.g., smoking cessation, stress management, substance misuse, or weight maintenance).

College/University Setting. Health educators in this setting may be involved in a variety of administrative responsibilities, including coordination of professional preparation programs and chairing of an academic department. Responsibilities might also include coordinating and supervising student internships and chairing or facilitating faculty or community committees.

University Health Services Setting. Health educators in the university health services setting may find themselves administering health education or health promotion programs, or in some cases, the health services center itself. In this role, the health educator must be able to plan and organize the program or center and administer both personnel and budgetary issues.

Area VI: Serve as a Health Education Resource Person

	Entry (Baccalaureate/master's, less than 5 years' experience)	**Advanced 1** (Baccalaureate/master's, 5 years' experience or more)	**Advanced 2** (Doctorate and 5 years' experience or more)
Competency A: Use health-related information resources	1. Match information needs with the appropriate retrieval systems 2. Select a data system commensurate with program needs 3. Determine the relevance of various computerized health information resources 4. Access health information resources 5. Employ electronic technology for retrieving references	. . .	. . .
Competency B: Respond to requests for health information	1. Identify information sources needed to satisfy a request 2. Refer requesters to valid sources of health information	. . .	. . .
Competency C: Select resource materials for dissemination	1. Evaluate applicability of resource materials for given audience 2. Apply various processes to acquire resource materials 3. Assemble educational material of value to the health of individuals and community groups	. . .	. . .
Competency D: Establish consultative relationships	1. Analyze parameters of effective consultative relationships 2. Analyze the role of the health educator as a liaison between program staff and outside groups and organizations 3. Act as a liaison among consumer groups, individuals, and health care provider organizations 4. Apply networking skills to develop and maintain consultative relationships 5. Facilitate collaborative training efforts among health agencies and organizations	. . .	1. Describe consulting skills needed by health educators

Area of Responsibility VI: Serve as a Health Education Resource Person

The Role. The setting in which the health educator functions largely determines the nature of the resources provided. When requested, health educators need to serve as a resource for valid health information. They must be aware of a variety of community resources, familiar with computer-based retrieval systems and national on-line databases, and skillful at locating valid information through Internet searches.

In addition, the health educator needs to be able to evaluate and select resource materials for dissemination to individuals and groups. Being a resource person also means that the health educator must be able to establish consultative relationships and develop the skills necessary for serving as a liaison, for networking, and for facilitating collaborative efforts.

Settings.

Community Setting. In the community setting, health educators might be asked to serve on county-wide drug abuse councils. They would make available data from research studies and best practices; recommend relevant literature; suggest audiovisual materials, educational pamphlets, and posters for distribution; and report on successful drug prevention and intervention programs being conducted elsewhere.

School (K-12) Setting. A health educator in the school setting might participate in the work of a curriculum committee formed to identify and select sexuality education materials that would be in compliance with state legislative mandates and school district policies. The health educator might be asked to assist committee members in examining state laws and codes, establishing criteria for the evaluation of such materials, and recommending placement of the topic in the overall curriculum scope and sequence plan. After selection of the material, the health educator might also arrange preview sessions for interested parents and community members.

Health Care Setting. A health educator in the health care setting might serve as a consultant to a community group in developing a cancer education program. The health educator would provide information on successful programs; help identify culturally and linguistically appropriate materials; conduct focus groups to assist in planning interventions; identify expert speakers; and help identify media and other communication channels for disseminating information about the program to the community.

Business/Industry Setting. Physical fitness programs are frequently featured in worksite health promotion programming. As a resource person, the health educator would be responsible for explaining to both employers and employees the costs and benefits of such programs. Health educators can identify and organize resources needed for the implementation and continuation of the fitness or other health promotion programs. They can identify research data to present to concerned personnel and monitor the plans of those responsible for conducting the program to ensure that its activities match the stated goals and objectives.

College/University Setting. The professor teaching a course in a health education professional preparation program might have students serve as consultants to a local school district as the district team members try to assess their Coordinated School Health Program using the School Health Index. As the students work with the local district they are sharpening their consulting and networking skills.

University Health Services Setting. The health educator in the university health services setting might establish a Web site where students and staff can obtain information about health-related topics such as nutrition and physical activity. The Web site should contain links to a number of sites containing current and reliable health information.

Area VII: Communicate and Advocate for Health and Health Education

	Entry (Baccalaureate/master's, less than 5 years' experience)	Advanced 1 (Baccalaureate/master's, 5 years' experience or more)	Advanced 2 (Doctorate and 5 years' experience or more)
Competency A: Analyze and respond to current and future needs in health education	1. Analyze factors (e.g., social, cultural, demographic, and political) that influence decision-makers	1. Respond to challenges facing health education programs 2. Implement strategies for advocacy initiatives 3. Use evaluation data to advocate for health education programs	1. Analyze the interrelationships among ethics, values, and behavior 2. Relate health education issues to larger social issues
Competency B: Apply a variety of communication methods and techniques	1. Assess the appropriateness of language in health education messages 2. Compare different methods of distributing educational materials 3. Respond to public input regarding health education information 4. Use culturally sensitive communication methods and techniques 5. Use appropriate techniques when communicating health and health education information 6. Use oral, electronic, and written techniques for communicating health education information 7. Demonstrate proficiency in communicating health information and health education needs	. . .	. . .
Competency C: Promote the health education profession individually and collectively	1. Develop a personal plan for professional growth	. . .	1. Describe the state of the art of health education practice 2. Explain the major responsibilities of the health educator in the practice of health education 3. Explain the role of health education associations in advancing the profession 4. Explain the benefits of participating in professional organizations
Competency D: Influence health policy to promote health	1. Identify the significance and implications of health care providers' messages to consumers	1. Use research results to develop health policy	1. Describe how research results influence health policy 2. Use evaluation findings in policy analysis and development

SECTION: III

Area of Responsibility VII: Communicate and Advocate for Health and Health Education

The Role. Health educators are charged with the responsibility to provide information to diverse audiences. Whether through individual, small group, or mass communication techniques, health educators use their professional background to interpret consumer needs and concerns. They also communicate to others the unique foundations of and contributions offered by health education professionals across a range of employment settings. To that end, health educators consider the value systems of the intended audience as well as an array of educational strategies best suited to communicating the required information.

Settings.

Community Setting. A health educator employed in a voluntary health organization with a volunteer board of directors might be charged with the responsibility of providing board members with information about current levels of community need for a particular program. The health educator would marshal appropriate data and present it to the board. The health educator would also provide information about consumer perspectives on the program to better equip the board in making an informed decision about the program's direction. Beyond small group discussions, the health educator might meet with individual board members to ensure that information is explained appropriately and is understood by all members, who may have diverse professional backgrounds.

School (K-12) Setting. When employed in a school setting, a health educator might be responsible for presenting curriculum information and student health information needs and concerns to groups of parents. In the event of parental concerns, the health educator would take into consideration the multiple value systems represented by the group and would employ appropriate strategies to communicate the material and respond to parents' questions. Depending upon the topic, the health educator might use illustrations from classroom instruction, student presentations, or videotapes to enhance the presentation.

Health Care Setting. In this setting, the health educator might be responsible for a program to support patients' smoking cessation efforts. The health educator would need to communicate with providers regarding the importance of the program, as well as the health educator's appropriateness for launching such an effort. With the providers' understanding and support, the health educator would be responsible for informing the priority population of the program's availability in ways consistent with the values of the intended audience. Brochures, posters, flyers, public service announcements, and various electronic media might be considered.

Business/Industry Setting. A health educator employed in the workplace might become aware of some previously unrecognized health need among workers. The health educator would communicate that need (e.g., insufficient opportunity for physical activity) to management. Using his or her background in behavioral and biological sciences, the health educator would interpret the problem for management and articulate the health educator's role in addressing it. Acknowledging concerns specific to management, the health educator could then communicate ways in which a health education program might benefit both management and the worker.

College/University Setting. A health educator in a college/university setting might be faced with the challenge of ensuring health education's place in the college curriculum. Recognizing that there are multiple perspectives on what constitutes an educated student, the health educator would consider colleagues' orientations and use that information in formulating presentations on the importance of health education in the university environment. This communication might be handled through reports to curriculum committees, presentations before administrators, or small group discussions with students and faculty.

University Health Services Setting. In a university health services setting, the health educator interfaces with students, health care providers, faculty, and parents. In that arena, the health educator might be charged with providing an educational program to improve students' decision making about use of drugs and alcohol. The health educator would communicate to health care providers the need for such a program, working with them to establish health education's contributions to such a program and to ensure the providers' support and participation. The health educator should be able to frame the effort in a way that offends neither parental nor student values. The health educator would communicate the educational purpose of the program to students and interpret its value relative to their health education needs and concerns. This communication could be handled through flyers given to individual students, posters placed around campus, and presentations before small groups within dormitories. The health educator might also work with sororities to encourage alternatives to alcohol consumption and advocate for local laws or ordinances that stiffen alcohol or drug-related offenses for businesses.

Section IV:
Using the CUP Model

Section IV: Using the CUP Model

The CUP Model provides universities, professional organizations, and accreditation agencies with a common set of competencies for the development, assessment, and improvement of professional preparation, credentialing procedures, and professional development for health educators. As in earlier versions, the CUP competencies and sub-competencies are considered generic and independent of the setting in which the health educator works. The CUP Model provides distinct sets of competencies and sub-competencies for the three levels of practice (i.e., Entry, Advanced 1, and Advanced 2).

In addition to assisting college and university faculty in health education curriculum development, the CUP Model will help to guide and inform health education students, practicing health educators, employers, accrediting bodies, policy makers, and others. The diffusion of the CUP model into professional preparation, credentialing, and professional development should underscore the value and benefits of using a competency-based approach to health education. Health educators are encouraged to discern useful and innovative ways to incorporate such an approach into their practice. While a health educator's work setting and stipulated work responsibilities will tend to direct his or her key practices, the CUP Model can serve as a helpful guide for the development of more comprehensive roles and responsibilities.

The Health Education Student

For the student or prospective student, the CUP Model, in keeping with earlier models, provides a look at the health education profession as defined by the seven areas of responsibility (see Table 1). Prospective students can use the CUP Model to determine whether the curriculum in a potential program of study will enable them to meet these health education responsibilities and their respective competencies and sub-competencies.

Once enrolled in an undergraduate or graduate health education program, students can use the CUP Model in the form of a personal inventory to assess progress toward becoming a health educator, that is, to determine which competencies and sub-competencies have been mastered. It might be helpful for students to assess their progress at different intervals during their course of study and conduct final reviews at the completion of their health education program. Thus, the CUP Model can be used as a self-assessment tool to identify opportunities to improve areas of weakness or to outline a potential career ladder and the courses needed to climb it.

College and University Faculty

The CUP Model has the potential to strengthen the curricula of professional preparation programs in health education throughout the United States. It can be used by college and university faculty to generate clearer expectations for student performance. Colleges and universities can also use the CUP Model to develop programs that specifically address deficits that students might have or as the foundation of a portfolio approach to student assessment.

The curriculum for the professional preparation of health educators would benefit from a competency-based approach. The CUP research results provide a nationally validated model that can be used as a standard of comparison for programs preparing health educators at the baccalaureate, master's, and doctoral levels. Periodically, faculty review curricula to determine relevance and currency or to meet nationally recognized standards (see Appendix D for matrices for analyzing curricula). The CUP Model will be useful in these reviews, and program revisions should address the sub-competencies and competencies within the seven areas of responsibility. Faculty are encouraged to assess the degree to which their curricula and other professional preparation opportunities meet the CUP Model prior to seeking program accreditation.

The Health Education Practitioner

The CUP Model can be used by the practitioner as a guide for professional growth and development. Health educators in the field can use the model as a guide in selecting continuing education opportunities that will enhance their skills and address their deficits in the seven areas of responsibility and their respective competencies and sub-competencies. Organizations involved in providing continuing education and professional development activities, such as professional societies, universities and state agencies, will need to consider aligning their efforts with the CUP Model so the new areas of responsibility, competencies, and sub-competencies identified by the CUP research will be addressed.

Other Health Professionals

Professionals outside health education often have a limited view of the specific skills and abilities of the health educator. The CUP Model can be used to enhance the understanding and appreciation of health education at all three levels of practice. Partnerships between professionals can be established by determining where the roles of disciplines overlap and where they depart from the roles of health educators, thereby maximizing collaborative efforts in the provision of services.

Health Education Employers

The CUP results will have significance for employers, who will now have updated expectations of the competencies that employees should possess, and for health educators, who will have clearer direction regarding current practice. It is important that employers be able to recognize the knowledge and skills that professionally prepared health educators can bring to the workplace. Emphasizing that these are empirically based skills should heighten the value of having qualified health education practitioners in a variety of work settings.

Employers in business and education are accustomed to seeking out the most qualified workers and should continue to look for those who possess the competencies necessary to successfully perform the job. In health education, the Certified Health Education Specialist (CHES) credential indicates mastery of the responsibilities, competencies, and sub-competencies identified by the profession. When seeking personnel for worksite health promotion, patient education, school health, and other health education programs, employers would be advised to use the CUP results in their job descriptions and position announcements.

Credentialing and the Certified Health Education Specialist

The CUP Model will impact credentialing processes, particularly individual certification and program accreditation, contributing to their validity and consistency. The model suggests the potential for additional certification processes at different levels of practice. In the course of the CUP research, statistically significant differences in the generic (i.e., across work settings) Entry-level and Advanced-level sub-competencies were found. While the Entry-level sub-competencies are considered "building blocks" for health educators at each level of practice, additional and more extensive sub-competencies are required at the Advanced levels. At the time the research was conducted, the national certification examination for the CHES credential was designed to assess one's competency solely at the Entry level. Now that validated sub-competencies have been identified at the two Advanced levels of practice, advanced levels of certification will undoubtedly be explored.

Policy Makers and Funding Agencies

The CUP Model can be used by policy makers at all levels of government (federal, state, and local), as well as policy makers in nongovernmental organizations, schools, and businesses, in

- Developing health programs
- Establishing organizational policies
- Considering community, state, or national policy (i.e., laws, regulation, and ordinances)
- Determining criteria for funding projects and individuals
- Educating boards, management, and leadership about the potential of health education

The model clarifies for policy makers the skills and competencies professionally prepared health educators should bring to a program or multidisciplinary team. In addition, it identifies those skills an entry-level professional should have versus an individual with more experience or a higher academic degree.

It is anticipated that various aspects of the CUP research and model will be valuable to public policy makers undertaking other projects related to quality assurance and credentialing of the public health workforce. The U.S. Department of Labor and the states are implementing the Standard Occupation Classification system, which now requires distinct data collection for the occupation of health educator. Clearly, the CUP research and model have important implications for workforce development and the professional development of the health educator.

Recommendations to the Profession

In 2005, the boards of SOPHE, AAHE, and NCHEC issued the following recommendations for using the CUP Model. The recommendations were endorsed in 2006 by the Coalition of National Health Education Organizations, whose members (in addition to AAHE and SOPHE) include representatives from American Academy of Health Behavior, American College Health Association, American Public Health Association (School Health Education and Services Section and the Public Health Education and Health Promotion Section), American School Health Association, Directors of Health Promotion and Education, Eta Sigma Gamma, and Society of State Directors of Health, Physical Education, and Recreation.

1. Baccalaureate programs in health education should prepare their health education graduates to perform all 7 of the health education responsibilities and the 29 competencies and 82 sub-competencies specifically identified as Entry-level in the new hierarchical model.

2. NCHEC should use all 7 of the health education responsibilities and the 29 competencies and 82 sub-competencies specifically identified as Entry-level in the new hierarchical model as the basis for revisions to its entry-level CHES examination.

3. Graduate programs in health education should prepare their health education graduates to perform all 7 of the health education responsibilities and the 48 Advanced 1 and 33 Advanced 2 sub-competencies as appropriate to the degree level. Advanced 1 and Advanced 2 graduates should also demonstrate mastery of the 29 Entry-level competencies and 82 Entry-level sub-competencies in the new hierarchical model.

4. When organizations interpret the CUP findings for use in professional preparation, credentialing, and professional development, a clear written rationale should accompany the interpretations being made. ◆

A Competency-Based Framework for Health Educators – 2006

Section V:
Changes in the Responsibilities, Competencies, and Sub-competencies of Health Educators From 1985 to 2006

Section V: Changes in the Responsibilities, Competencies, and Sub-competencies of Health Educators From 1985 to 2006

SECTION: V

More than 20 years have passed since the role of entry-level health educators and their related scope of practice was articulated in the basic seven areas of responsibility. For the most part, the areas of responsibility in the CUP Model are not profoundly different from those original seven, which is a testament to the solid foundations on which the profession stands. Yet the CUP research did reveal substantial changes in, and the emergence of, a variety of new competencies and sub-competencies. These updated competencies and sub-competencies not only reflect dramatic social, technological, demographic, and other trends in recent decades, but also significant maturation of the health education profession in terms of a more robust level of theory and practice.

The dynamic CUP Model will undoubtedly impact many sectors involved in health education, not least of which are professional preparation, credentialing, and continuing education. The hierarchical nature of the CUP Model (i.e., all competencies at the Entry level are expected to be mastered by health educators at the Advanced 1 level and all competencies at the Entry and Advanced 1 levels are expected to be mastered by those at the Advanced 2 level) also is expected to significantly alter the way graduate faculty approach curriculum development and revision as well as practitioners' self-assessments and plans for lifelong learning.

Seven Areas of Responsibility

The most obvious change in the CUP Model is the return to seven areas of responsibility from the ten areas found in the 1999 framework for graduate-level health educators. The original seven, developed in the early 1980s, were designated as Entry level and have served as the basis of the individual credentialing process. Three additional areas of responsibility were added for the post-baccalaureate health educator in the late 1990s; those areas have now been integrated within the seven areas of responsibility in the CUP Model.

Area of Responsibility I, Assess Individual and Community Need for Health Education, has been expanded. The number of competencies has increased from three (four at the graduate level) to six. This change reflects the need for more data collection, manipulation, and analysis skills at the Entry level than were necessary two decades ago.

Area of Responsibility II, Plan Health Education Strategies, Interventions, and Programs, has been expanded from four competencies (five at the post-baccalaureate level) to seven and has been modified to reflect the scope of practice of the health educator. There is a shift of competencies between Entry and Advanced 1 levels, with the Entry-level health educator having more data collection and program implementation responsibilities than in prior years, while the Advanced 1 professional is expected to be more proficient in program design. In addition, the Advanced 2 health educator is expected to demonstrate significant competencies in the use of theory in designing programs, strategies, and interventions.

Area of Responsibility III, Implement Health Education Strategies, Interventions, and Programs, continues to include four competencies, but these competencies and sub-competencies have been revised to more directly address the skills necessary for program implementation. In addition, ethics has moved from graduate level to Entry level, recognizing the importance of an ethical foundation for health education practice.

Area of Responsibility IV, Conduct Evaluation and Research Related to Health Education, is a synthesis of areas of responsibility IV and VIII of the 1999 graduate-level model. More responsibility for research and evaluation has migrated to the Entry level, while the Advanced 1 professional is now expected to focus on the implementation of findings.

Area of Responsibility V, Administer Health Education Strategies, Interventions, and Programs, replaces the former area of responsibility V with a new administrative responsibility more closely aligned with area of responsibility IX of the 1999 graduate-level model. This responsibility lies almost exclusively at the Advanced 1 level, as the administrative function tends to occur after experience is gained. Many of the coordination functions included in the former area of responsibility V have migrated to other areas of responsibility.

Area of Responsibility VI, Serve as a Health Education Resource Person, is heavily weighted toward knowledge and skills expected for Entry-level practitioners. This responsibility uses the most basic skills of the Health Educator and its importance cannot be overstated. Thus, it is necessary that this area of responsibility be mastered at the Entry level and then carried over into the Advanced 1 and Advanced 2 levels.

Area of Responsibility VII, Communicate and Advocate for Health and Health Education, has changed appreciably from the old area of responsibility VII. While communication remains the primary focus of the Entry level, Advanced levels 1 and 2 both strongly support the concept of the health educator as advocate. This change indicates a new role for health educators in impacting policy change that must be acknowledged.

Two Advanced Levals

A second major change from the former entry- and graduate-level health education models is the division of the advanced level of training into two categories, Advanced 1 and Advanced 2. Both Entry-level and Advanced 1 health educators may have either a baccalaureate or a master's degree; the difference is in length of experience. Health educators at the Entry level have less than five years' experience, while those at the Advanced 1 level have five years' experience or more. Advanced 2 is a completely new concept, entailing both a higher degree (doctorate) and more experience.

The Advanced 2 health educator reflects health education's grounding in real-world practice coupled with formal preparation. This level also speaks to the profession's exciting potential for career mobility, with opportunities to extend and refine our role as we contribute to the profession. As the most recently acknowledged level, however, Advanced 2 is also the least understood, because fewer data are available on the health educator's role at this level. Hence observations about the current and projected roles for those with such an educational and experiential background must be made cautiously.

Health educators at the Advanced 2 level appear to function in a manner consistent with their extensive experience and education. Their expertise is evident in terms of their responsibilities relative to the conduct of health education, to other health educators, and to the broader landscape in which we practice. For example, with respect to the conduct of health education programs, the Advanced 2 health educator has the major responsibilities in linking theory and practice. Whether in selecting educational materials or determining intervention strategies, the Advanced 2 health educator often works with colleagues to link theory and standards of best practice to program development and implementation. When evaluating programs, the Advanced 2 health educator brings breadth and depth to the evaluation process, working to select, apply, and interpret realistic quantitative and qualitative approaches in meaningful ways.

While all health educators have responsibilities to each other, the Advanced 2 is most likely to act as a mentor to other health educators. More than their colleagues at the other levels, Advanced 2 health educators assume responsibility for securing fiscal resources and supporting those who deliver professional development. They are among the profession's own teachers, applying instructional resources to diverse training needs. They also are most likely to serve as faculty of health education preparation programs as well as interface with those curious about the profession. As such, Advanced 2 health educators have the ability to spark interest among those unfamiliar with health education, to encourage their consideration of the profession, and to help perpetuate the profession's vitality. In so doing, Advanced 2 health educators' mentor role extends beyond the classroom to include such behaviors as informing their less experienced colleagues of the benefits of membership in professional organizations.

Finally, the Advanced 2 health educator promises, perhaps more than others in the field, to develop as a spokesperson for health and health education. Advanced 2 health educators have the critical and often daunting task of explaining health educators' contributions in terms of the larger social, behavioral, and ethical contexts in which they work. Their voices promote the profession by describing what it is that they do and how their findings and programs influence health policy. They also are the health educators charged with looking to the future. With the combined strength of their practice and educational bases, Advanced 2 health educators anticipate health education needs as well as the social context in which those needs must be met and potential obstacles to their being met.

This section highlights the most notable differences between the new CUP Model, which reflects the scope of practice of the health educator in the 21st century, and its predecessors. For a more detailed comparison of the CUP Model with the previous models, see Appendix B. ◆

References:

References

Allegrante, J.P., Airhihenbuwa, C.O., Auld, M.E., Birch, D.A., Roe, K.M., Smith, B.J. (2004). Toward a Unified System of Accreditation for Professional Preparation in Health Education: Final Report of the National Task Force on Accreditation in Health Education. *Health Education & Behavior, 31*(6), 668-683.

American Association for Health Education (2005). Directory of institutions offering undergraduate and graduate degree programs in health education. *American Journal of Health Education, 36*(6), 345-360.

American Association for Health Education (AAHE), National Commission for Health Education Credentialing (NCHEC), & Society for Public Health Education (SOPHE). (1999). *A competency-based framework for graduate-level health educators.* Allentown, PA: NCHEC.

Cleary, H.P. (1995). *The credentialing of health educators: An historical account, 1970-1990.* Allentown, PA: NCHEC.

Cleary, H.P. (1997). The credentialing of health educators: An historical account, 1970-1990. *CHES Bulletin, 8*(1), 11-19.

Coalition of National Health Education Organizations (CNHEO). (1999). *Code of ethics for the health education profession.* Available from: http://www.hsc.usf.edu/CFH/cnheo/downloads/code2.pdf.

Gilmore, G.D., Olsen, L.K., & Taub, A. (2001). *Competencies update project: Promoting quality assurance in health education.* Rockville, MD: Bureau of Health Professions, Health Resources and Services Administration.

Gilmore, G.D., Olsen, L.K., & Taub, A. (2004). *National health educator competencies update project, 1998-2004: Technical report.* Allentown, PA: AAHE, NCHEC, and SOPHE.

Gilmore, G.D., Olsen, L.K., Taub, A., & Connell, D. (2004). *The National Health Educator Competencies Update Project: Research process and methodological innovations/insights.* Silver Spring, MD: Report prepared for the Agency for Healthcare Research and Quality.

Gilmore, G.D., Olsen, L.K., Taub, A., & Connell, D. (2005). Overview of the National Health Educator Competencies Update Project, 1998-2004. *Health Education & Behavior, 32(6):725-737.*

Henderson, A.C., & McIntosh, D.V. (August 22, 1981). *Role refinement and verification for entry-level health educators.* (HRP-0904273). Springfield, VA: National Technical Information Service.

Joint Committee on Health Education and Promotion Terminology. (2001). Report of the 2000 Joint Committee on Health Education and Promotion Terminology. *American Journal of Health Education, 32(20)*, 89-104.

Linacre, J.M. (1998). *A user's guide to Facets: Rasch measurement computer program.* Chicago: MESA.

Linacre, J.M. (1999). Facets (Version 3.1) [computer software]. Chicago: MESA.

Linacre, J. (2003). *A user's guide to FACETS: Rasch-model computer programs.* Chicago: Winsteps (http://www.winsteps.com).

Livingood, W.C., Auld, M.E. (2001). The credentialing of a population-based profession: lessons learned from health education certification. *Journal of Public Health Management & Practice, 7(4)*, 38-45.

National Commission for Health Education Credentialing (NCHEC). (1985). *A framework for the development of competency-based curricula for entry-level health educators.* New York: Author.

National Commission for Health Education Credentialing (NCHEC). (1990). *Recertification handbook for CHES.* New York: Author.

National Commission for Health Education Credentialing (NCHEC). (1996). A *competency-based framework for professional development of certified health education specialists.* Allentown, PA: Author.

Neutens, J. (1984). Professional Competencies of the Health Educator. In L. Rubinson & W. Alles (Eds.), *Health Education Foundations for the Future.* Prospect Heights, IL: Waveland Press.

Rasch G. (1990). *Probabilistic models for some intelligence and attainment tests.* Chicago: MESA.

Schulman, J.A., Trujillo, M.J., & Karney, B.R. (2001). Facets: Computer software for evaluating assessment tools. *American Journal of Health Behavior, 25(1)*, 75-77.

Society for Public Health Education (SOPHE) & American Association for Health Education (AAHE). (1997). *Standards for the preparation of graduate-level health educators.* Washington, DC: Author.

U.S. Department of Health, Education and Welfare, Health Resources Administration, Bureau of Health Manpower. (1978). *Preparation and practice of community, patient, and school health educators: Proceedings of the Workshop on Commonalities and Differences.* Washington, DC: Division of Allied Health Professions.

REFERENCES

Appendices

Glossary

The glossary explains terms used in this document. These definitions are not all-inclusive but are intended to convey the meaning of terms within the context of this document.

Advanced level 1 – The level of a health educator with a baccalaureate or a master's degree and five years' experience or more in the field of health education.

Advanced level 2 – The level of a health educator with a doctoral degree and five years' experience or more in the field of health education.

Area of responsibility – One of the major categories of performance expectations of a proficient health education practitioner. The areas of responsibility define the scope of practice (SOPHE & AAHE, 1997).

Certified Health Education Specialist (CHES) – An individual who has met required health education training qualifications, has successfully passed a competency-based examination administered by the National Commission for Health Education Credentialing, Inc., and satisfies the continuing education requirement to maintain the national credential (Joint Committee on Health Education and Promotion Terminology, 2001).

Credentialing – An umbrella term referring to the various means employed to designate that individuals or organizations have met or exceeded established standards. These standards may include certification, registration, or licensure of individuals or accreditation of organizations. Health education has chosen certification as the method of individual credentialing for the profession (NCHEC, n.d.).

Coalition – An alliance, often temporary, that allows two or more groups or organizations to promote a common cause (AAHE, NCHEC, & SOPHE, 1999).

Competency – A broadly defined skill or ability, adequate performance of which is expected of the health educator. Mastery of a competency is dependent upon achievement of clusters of simpler but essential related skills or abilities (NCHEC, 1990).

Entry level – The level of a health educator with a baccalaureate or master's degree and less than five years' experience in the field of health education.

APEND. A

Health education – Any combination of planned learning experiences based on sound theories that provide individuals, groups, and communities the opportunity to acquire the information and skills needed to make quality health decisions (Joint Committee on Health Education and Promotion Terminology, 2001).

Health educator – A professionally prepared individual who serves in a variety of roles and is specifically trained to use appropriate educational strategies and methods to facilitate the development of policies, procedures, interventions, and systems conducive to the health of individuals, groups, and communities (Joint Committee on Health Education and Promotion Terminology, 2001).

Health literacy – The capacity of an individual to obtain, interpret, and understand basic health information and services and the competence to use such information and services in ways that are health enhancing (Joint Committee on Health Education and Promotion Terminology, 2001).

Profession – A group of individuals with similar educational preparation who come together for a common occupational goal and that usually exhibits the following characteristics: (1) provides a unique and essential service; (2) requires of its members an extensive period of preparation; (3) has a theoretical base underlying its practice; (4) has a system of internal controls, including a code of ethics that tends to regulate the behavior of its members; (5) has a culture peculiar to the profession; 6) is sanctioned by the community; and (7) has an occupational association representative of and able to speak on behalf of all members of the profession (Neutens, 1984).

Professional development – Planned learning activities designed to maintain and enhance one's competence in health education following a previously attained level of professional preparation (Joint Committee on Health Education and Promotion Terminology, 2001).

Professional preparation – An undergraduate or graduate course of study that includes career-related experiences offered through an accredited college or university, which is designed to prepare individuals to practice competently in the health education field (Joint Committee on Health Education and Promotion Terminology, 2001).

Standard – The predetermined level of performance at which a criterion will be considered met. If a desired condition or characteristic (e.g., curricular content that assures development of specific health education competencies) is the criterion, the standard then expresses the minimum acceptable content that will satisfy the expectation (NCHEC, 1999).

APEND. A

Comparison of the Areas of Responsibilty, Competencies, and Sub-competencies of the 1999 Framework with the CUP Model

As part of the overall development of this document, and to make it more valuable to the user, an individual item analysis of the 1999 framework (which contained the entry- and graduate-level model, herein denoted "Old") and the CUP Model (denoted "New") was conducted. This analysis, conducted by a subcommittee from the Division Board for Certification of Health Education Specialists of the National Commission for Health Education Credentialing, Inc., highlights additions, removals, and changes in placement of areas of responsibility, competencies, and sub-competencies. This analysis can be used by various segments of the profession to adapt the new information to professional preparation, credentialing, and professional development.

The comparison of the old and new areas of responsibility, competencies, and sub-competencies that follows is a result of a multi-step process of individual and then group reviews, shared insights, and reevaluation to very carefully examine the differences and similarities and reach a consensus. The placement and wording of the competencies is based on the CUP research and could not be altered. During the analysis it became apparent that many of the items in the new model are similar to items in the previous version but reworded or refined. For the purpose of this analysis, the determination is based on the literal wording, rather than attempting to interpret the intent.

The review that resulted in this comparison chart was first created for the purpose of exam realignment; it can be used for curriculum design as well. The limitation of this analysis is that it is based on wording alone, not intent. Therefore, this analysis should be used as a guide; determinations of actual impact on applications such as curriculum changes, exam construction, or continuing education will have to be tailored to the specific activity.

Several of the competencies and sub-competencies carried over from the old model have been placed in a different area of responsibility in the new model. This is particularly true of those previously in the graduate-level areas of responsibility VIII, IX, and X. Also of note, some items previously identified as entry-level are now reflected in one of the advanced levels and some items previously considered graduate-level have been moved to entry level.

Each item in the comparison chart has been classified as "NEW" (not in 1999 framework) or "LOSS" (in 1999 framework but not in the CUP model) or identified with a placement number showing its placement in the other model. The chart is placed in numerical order based on the new Competencies.

Comparison of the Areas of Responsibility, Competencies, and Sub-competencies of the 1999 Framework (OLD) with the National Health Educator Competencies Update Project (CUP) Model (NEW)

OLD		Sub-competencies		NEW		Entry (Baccalaureate/Master's, Less Than 5 Years' Experience)	Advanced 1 (Baccalaureate/Master's, 5 Years' Experience or More)	Advanced 2 (Doctorate and 5 Years' Experience or More)
Area of Responsibility I: Assessing Individual and Community Needs for Health Education				**Area of Responsibility I: Assess Individual and Community Needs for Health Education**				
I. Competency A: Obtain health-related data about social and cultural environments, growth and development factors, needs, and interests.	I.A AND I.B			**I. Competency A:** Access existing health-related data.	I.A			
		I.A.1. Select valid sources of information about health needs and interests.	I.A.E.4	I.A.E.1. Identify diverse health-related databases.		NEW		
								I.A.A2.1. Critique sources of health information. — VIII.A.3
		I.A.2. Utilize computerized sources of health-related information.	I.A.E.2	I.A.E.2. Use computerized sources of health-related information.		I.A.2		
		I.A.3. Employ or develop appropriate data-gathering instruments.	IV.C.E.2 & I.B.E.1	I.A.E.3. Determine the compatibility of data from different data sources.		NEW		
		I.A.4. Apply survey techniques to acquire health data.	I.B.E.2	I.A.E.4. Select valid sources of information about health needs and interests.		I.A.1		
		I.A.5. Conduct health-related needs assessment in communities.	TO ENTRY I.B.E.3	**I. Competency B:** Collect health-related data.	I.A			
				I.B.E.1. Use appropriate data-gathering instruments.		I.A.3		
				I.B.E.2. Apply survey techniques to acquire health data.		I.A.4		
				I.B.E.3. Conduct health-related needs assessments.		I.A.5.		
				I.B.E.4. Implement appropriate measures to assess capacity for improving health status.		NEW		
I. Competency B: Distinguish between behaviors that foster and those that hinder well-being.	I.C			**I. Competency C:** Distinguish between behaviors that foster or hinder well-being.	I.B			
		I.B.1. Investigate physical, social, emotional and intellectual factors influencing health behaviors.	I.C.E.1	I.C.E.1. Identify diverse factors that influence health behaviors.		I.B.1		
		I.B.2. Identify behaviors that tend to promote or compromise health.	I.C.E.2	I.C.E.2. Identify behaviors that tend to promote or compromise health.		I.B.2		
		I.B.3. Recognize the role of learning and affective experience in shaping patterns of health behavior.	I.C.A.1.1				I.C.A1.1. Explain the role of experiences in shaping patterns of health behavior. — I.B.3	

Shaded area denotes graduate level competencies

APEND. B

OLD	Sub-competences	LOSS	NEW	Entry (Baccalaureate/Master's, Less Than 5 Years' Experience)	Advanced 1 (Baccalaureate/Master's, 5 Years' Experience or More)	Advanced 2 (Doctorate and 5 Years' Experience or More)
	I.B.4. Analyze social, cultural, economic, and political factors that influence health.	LOSS	NEW			
			I. Competency D: Determine factors that influence learning.		I.D.A1.1. Assess learning literacy. — New; I.D.A1.2. Assess learning styles. — New	I.D.A2.1. Assess the learning environment. — New
			NEW — **I. Competency E: Identify factors that foster or hinder the process of health education.**	I.E.E.1. Determine the extent of available health education services. — V.A.1; I.E.E.2. Identify gaps and overlaps in the provision of collaborative health services. — V.A.3	I.E.A1.1. Assess the environmental and political climate (e.g., organizational, community, state, and national) regarding conditions that advance or inhibit program goals. — IX.C.2	I.E.A2.1. Investigate social forces causing opposing viewpoints regarding health education needs and concerns. — VII.B.1
I. Competency C: Infer needs for health education on the basis of obtained data. (I.F)	I.C.1. Analyze needs assessment data. (LOSS: I.F.E.1) ; I.C.2. Determine priority areas of need for health education. (To Advance I.F.A1.1)		I.C — **I. Competency F: Infer needs for health education from obtained data.**	I.F.E.1. Analyze needs assessment data. — I.C.1	I.F.A1.1. Determine priorities for health education. — I.C.2	I.F.A2.1. Predict future health education needs based upon societal changes. — VII.B.4

Area of Responsibility II: Planning Effective Health Education Programs (OLD)

Area of Responsibility II: Plan Health Education Strategies, Interventions and Programs (NEW)

OLD	Sub-competences	LOSS	NEW	Entry (Baccalaureate/Master's, Less Than 5 Years' Experience)	Advanced 1 (Baccalaureate/Master's, 5 Years' Experience or More)	Advanced 2 (Doctorate and 5 Years' Experience or More)
II. Competency A: Recruit community organizations, resource people and potential participants for support and assistance in program planning. (II.A)	II.A.1. Communicate need for the program to those who will be involved. (II.B.E.4)		II.A — **II. Competency A: Involve people and organizations in program planning.**	II.A.E.1. Identify populations for health education programs. — NEW	II.A.A1.1. Involve participants in planning health education programs. — II.A.3	
	II.A.2. Obtain commitments from personnel and decision makers who will be involved in the program. (II.A.E.3)			II.A.E.2. Elicit input from those who will affect, or be affected by, the program. — II.A.3		
	II.A.3. Seek ideas and opinions of those who will affect, or be affected by, the program. (II.A.E.2)			II.A.E.3. Obtain commitments from individuals who will be involved in the program. — II.A.2		
	II.A.4. Incorporate feasible ideas and recommendations into the planning process. (LOSS)			II.A.E.4. Develop plans for promoting collaborative efforts among health agencies and organizations with mutual interests. — V.C.3		
	II.A.5. Apply principles of community organization in planning programs. (To Entry II.B.E.2)		NEW — **II. Competency B: Incorporate data analysis and principles of community organization.**	II.B.E.1. Use research results when planning programs. — VIII.C.2 ; II.B.E.2. Apply principles of community organization when planning programs. — II.A.5	II.B.A1.1. Incorporate results of needs assessment into the planning process. — NEW	

Shaded area denotes graduate level competencies

OLD		Sub-competencies		NEW		Entry (Baccalaureate/Master's, Less Than 5 Years' Experience)		Advanced 1 (Baccalaureate/Master's, 5 Years' Experience or More)		Advanced 2 (Doctorate and 5 Years' Experience or More)	
II. Competency C: Formulate appropriate and measurable program objectives.	II.C			II. Competency C: Formulate appropriate and measurable program objectives.	II.C	II.B.E.3. Suggest approaches for integrating health education within existing health programs.	V.C.2				
		II.C.1. Infer educational objectives that facilitate achievement of specified competencies.	LOSS			II.B.E.4. Communicate need for the program to those who will be involved.	II.A.1	II.C.A1.1. Establish criteria for health education program objectives.	NEW	II.C.A2.1. Develop subordinate measurable objectives as needed for instruction.	III.B.2
						II.C.E.1. Design developmentally appropriate interventions.	NEW (Refer II.C.1 & II.C.2)	II.C.A1.2. Develop program objectives based upon identified needs.	New		
		II.C.2. Develop a framework of broadly stated, operational objectives relevant to proposed health education program.	LOSS					II.C.A1.3. Appraise appropriateness of resources and materials relative to given objectives.	III.D.4	II.C.A2.2. Evaluate the efficacy of various methods to achieve objectives.	III.C.2
								II.C.A1.4. Revise program objectives as necessitated by changing needs.	NEW		
		II.B.1. Determine the range of health information requisite to a given program of instruction.	II.D.E.1	II. Competency D: Develop a logical scope and sequence plan for health education practice.	II.B	II.D.E.1. Determine the range of health information necessary for a given program of instruction.	II.B.1	II.D.A1.1. Organize the scope of the subject areas comprising the scope of a program in logical sequence.	II.B.2	II.D.A2.1. Incorporate theory-based foundations in planning health education programs.	II.B.5
		II.B.2. Organize the subject areas comprising the scope of a program in logical sequence.	To Advanced II.D.A1.1			II.D.E.2. Select references relevant to health education issues or programs.	VIII.A.2				
		II.B.3. Review philosophical and theory-based foundations in planning health education programs.	LOSS								
		II.B.4. Analyze the process for integrating health education as part of a broader health care or education program.	II.D.A1.2					II.D.A1.2. Analyze the process for integrating health education into other programs.	II.B.4		
		II.B.5 Develop a theory-based framework for health education programs.	II.D.A2.1								
II. Competency D: Design educational programs consistent with specified	II.E	II.D.1. Match proposed learning activities with those implicit in the stated objectives.	To Advanced II.E.A2.2	II. Competency E: Design strategies, interventions, and programs	II.D			II.E.A1.1. Plan a sequence of learning opportunities that reinforce mastery of	II.D.4	II.E.A2.1. Formulate a variety of educational methods.	II.D.2

Shaded area denotes graduate level competencies

APEND. B

OLD	Sub-competencies		NEW	Entry (Baccalaureate/Master's, Less Than 5 Years' Experience)		Advanced 1 (Baccalaureate/Master's, 5 Years' Experience or More)		Advanced 2 (Doctorate and 5 Years' Experience or More)	
program objectives.			consistent with specified objectives.			preceding objectives.			
	II.D.2. Formulate a wide variety of alternative educational methods.	To Advanced II.E.A2.1							
	II.D.3. Select strategies best suited to implementation of education objectives in a given setting.	To Advanced II.E.A1.2						II.E.A2.2. Match proposed learning activities with stated program objectives.	II.D.1
	II.D.4. Plan a sequence of learning opportunities building upon and reinforcing mastery of preceding objectives.	Advanced II.E.A1.1				II.E.A1.2. Select strategies best suited to achieve objectives in a given setting.	II.D.3		
	II.D.5. Select appropriate theory-based strategies in health program planning.	II.E.A2.3						II.E.A2.3. Select appropriate theory-based strategies in health program planning.	II.D.5
	II.D.6. Plan training and instructional programs for health professionals.	LOSS							
			II. Competency F: Select appropriate strategies to meet objectives.	II.F.E.1. Analyze technologies, methods, and media for their acceptability to diverse groups.	III.C.4 / II.D.3	II.F.A1.1. Plan training and instructional programs for diverse populations.	NEW	II.F.A2.1. Select educational materials consistent with accepted theory.	NEW
				II.F.E.2. Match health education services to proposed program activities.	V.A.2	II.F.A1.2. Incorporate communication strategies into program planning.	NEW		
			II. Competency G: Assess factors that affect implementation.	II.G.E.1. Determine the availability of information and resources needed to implement health education programs for a given audience.	NEW / III.C.3	II.G.A1.1. Analyze factors (e.g., learner characteristics, legal aspects, feasibility) that influence choices among implementation methods.	III.C.1.		
				II.G.E.2. Identify barriers to the implementation of health education programs.	NEW	II.G.A1.2. Select implementation strategies based upon research results.	VIII.C.3		
II. Competency E: Develop health education programs using social marketing principles.	II.E.1 Identify populations for health education programs.	To Entry II.A.E.1							
	II.E.2. Involve participants in planning health education programs.	To Entry II.A.A1.1							
	II.E.3 Design a marketing plan to promote health education.	LOSS							

Area of Responsibility III: Implementing Health Education Programs

Area of Responsibility III: Implement Health Education Strategies, Interventions, and Programs

Shaded area denotes graduate level competencies

APEND. B

Entry-Level Competency	(cross-ref)	Graduate-Level Competency	(cross-ref)	(Baccalaureate/Master's, Less Than 5 Years' Experience)	(code)	(Baccalaureate/Master's, 5 Years or More Experience)	(code)	Experience or More	(code)	Experience or More
III. Competency A: Exhibit competence in carrying out planned educational programs.	LOSS	**III. Competency A: Initiate a plan of action.**	NEW			III.A.A1.1. Apply individual or group process methods as appropriate to given learning situations.	III.A.2			
III.A.1. Employ a wide range of educational methods and techniques.	To Advanced III.B.A2.1	III.A.E.1. Use community organization principles to facilitate change conducive to health.			III.A.8					
III.A.2. Apply individual or group process methods as appropriate to given learning situations.	To Advanced III.A.A1.1	III.A.E.2. Pretest learners to determine baseline data relative to proposed program objectives.			III.B.1					
III.A.3. Utilize instructional equipment and other instructional media.	III.B.E.1	III.A.E.3. Deliver educational programs to diverse populations.			NEW					
III.A.4. Select methods that best facilitate the practice of program objectives.	To Advanced III.B.A1.1	III.A.E.4. Facilitate groups.			NEW (Refer Grad Comp V.C.4)					
III.A.5. Assess, select and apply technologies that will contribute to program objectives.	III.B.A.1.2									
III.A.6. Develop, demonstrate and model implementation strategies.	LOSS									
III.A.7. Deliver educational programs for health professionals.	LOSS									
III.A.8. Use community organization principles to guide and facilitate community development.	III.A.E.1									
III. Competency B: Infer enabling objectives as needed to implement instructional programs in specified settings.	LOSS	**III. Competency B: Demonstrate a variety of skills in delivering strategies, interventions, and programs.**	NEW	III.B.E.1. Use instructional technology effectively.	III.A.3	III.B.A1.1. Select methods that best facilitate achievement of program objectives.	III.A.4	III.B.A2.1. Use a variety of educational methods.	III.A.1	
III.B.1. Pretest learners to ascertain present abilities and knowledge relative to proposed program objectives.	III.A.E.2	III.B.E.2. Apply implementation strategies.			NEW	III.B.A1.2. Apply technologies that will contribute to program objectives.	NEW (Refer III.A.5)			
III.B.2. Develop subordinate measurable objectives as needed for instruction.	To Advanced III.C.A2.1									
III. Competency C: Select methods and media best suited to implement program plans for specific learners.		**III. Competency C: Use a variety of methods to implement strategies, interventions, and programs.**	NEW	III.C.E.1. Use the Code of Ethics in professional practice.	X.C.3	III.C.A1.1. Employ appropriate strategies when dealing with controversial health issues.	VII.B.2.			
III.C.1. Analyze learner characteristics, legal aspects, feasibility, and other considerations influencing choices among methods.	To Advanced II.G.A1.1	III.C.E.2. Apply theoretical and conceptual models from health education and related disciplines to improve program delivery.			III.C.5					
III.C.2. Evaluate the efficacy of alternative methods and techniques capable of facilitating program objectives.	To Advanced II.C.A2.2									

Shaded area denotes graduate level competencies

APEND. B

OLD	Sub-competencies		NEW	Entry (Baccalaureate/Master's, Less Than 5 Years' Experience)		Advanced 1 (Baccalaureate/Master's, 5 Years' Experience or More)		Advanced 2 (Doctorate and 5 Years' Experience or More)	
	III.C.3. Determine the availability of information, personnel, time, and equipment needed to implement the program for a given audience.	II.G.E.1	NEW	III.C.E.3. Demonstrate skills needed to develop capacity for improving health status.	NEW				
	III.C.4. Critically analyze technologies, methods, and media for their acceptability to diverse groups.	To Entry II.F.E.1		III.C.E.4. Incorporate demographically and culturally sensitive techniques when promoting programs.	IX.D.3				
	III.C.5. Apply theoretical and conceptual models from health education and related disciplines to improve program delivery.	To Entry III.C.E.2		III.C.E.5. Implement intervention strategies to facilitate health-related change.	NEW				
III. Competency D: Monitor educational programs, adjusting objectives and activities as necessary.	LOSS		III. Competency D: Conduct training programs.						
	III.D.1. Compare actual program activities with the stated objectives.	To Advanced IV.E.A1.1	V.D			III.D.A1.1. Demonstrate a wide range of strategies for conducting training programs.	V.D.3	III.D.A2.1. Use instructional resources that meet a variety of training needs.	V.D.2
	III.D.2. Assess the relevance of existing program objectives to current needs.	To Advanced IV.D.A1.1							
	III.D.3. Revise program activities and objectives as necessitated by changes in learner needs.	LOSS (refer II.C.A1.4)							
	III.D.4. Appraise applicability of resources and materials relative to given educational objectives.	To Advanced II.C.A1.3.							

Area of Responsibility IV: Evaluating Effectiveness of Health Education Programs / **Area of Responsibility IV: Conduct Evaluation and Research Related to Health Education**

OLD	Sub-competencies		NEW	Entry		Advanced 1		Advanced 2	
IV. Competency A: Develop plans to assess achievement of program objectives.	LOSS		IV. Competency A: Develop plans for evaluation and research.						
	IV.A.1. Determine standards of performance to be applied as criteria of effectiveness.	To Advanced IV.B.A.1.1	NEW	IV.A.E.1. Synthesize information presented in the literature.	VII.A.5				
	IV.A.2. Establish a realistic scope of evaluation efforts.	To Advanced IV.B.A2.1							
	IV.A.3. Develop an inventory of existing valid and reliable tests and instruments.	To Advanced IV.A.A1.1				IV.A.A1.1. Develop an inventory of existing valid and reliable tests and survey instruments.	IV.A.3	IV.A.A2.1. Assess the merits and limitations of qualitative and quantitative methods.	VIII.B.1
	IV.A.4. Select appropriate methods for evaluating program effectiveness.	To Advanced IV B.A1.3							
	IV.A.5. Identify existing sources of health-related databases.	To Entry I.A.E.1		IV.A.E.2. Evaluate research designs, methods, and	VIII.A.4				

Shaded area denotes graduate level competencies

OLD	Sub-competencies		NEW	Entry (Baccalaureate/Master's, Less Than 5 Years' Experience)		Advanced 1 (Baccalaureate/Master's, 5 Years' Experience or More)		Advanced 2 (Doctorate and 5 Years' Experience or More)	
	IV.A.6. Evaluate existing data-gathering instruments and processes.	To Entry IV.B.E.1			findings presented in the literature.				
	IV.A.7. Select appropriate qualitative and/or qualitative evaluation design.	IV.B.A2.2							
	IV.A.8. Develop valid and reliable evaluation instruments.	To Entry IV.C.E.1							
			IV. Competency B: Review research and evaluation procedures.	NEW	IV.B.E.1. Evaluate data-gathering instruments and processes. [IV.A.6]	IV.A.1	IV.B.A.1.1. Identify standards of performance to be applied as criteria of effectiveness.	IV.A.2	IV.B.A2.1. Establish a realistic scope of evaluation efforts.
				NEW	IV.B.E.2. Develop methods to evaluate factors that influence shifts in health status.	NEW	IV.B.A1.2. Identify methods to evaluate factors that influence shifts in health status.	IV.A.7	
						IV.A.4	IV.B.A1.3. Select appropriate methods for evaluating program effectiveness.		IV.B.A2.2. Select appropriate qualitative and/or quantitative evaluation design.
			IV. Competency C: Design data collection instruments.	I.A.3	IV.C.E.1. Develop valid and reliable evaluation instruments. [IV.A.8]				
				NEW	IV.C.E.2. Develop appropriate data-gathering instruments.				
IV. Competency B: Carry out evaluation plans.	IV.D		**IV. Competency D: Carry out evaluation and research plans.**	NEW	IV.D.E.1. Use appropriate research methods and designs in health education practice.	III.D.2	IV.D.A1.1. Assess the relevance of existing program objectives to current needs.	IV.B.5	IV.D.A2.1. Apply appropriate evaluation technology.
	IV.B.1. Facilitate administration of the tests and activities specified in the plan.	To Advanced V.A.A2.1							
	IV.B.2. Utilize data-collecting methods appropriate to the objectives.	IV.D.E.2		IV.B.2	IV.D.E.2. Use data collection methods appropriate for measuring stated objectives.			NEW (Refer IV.C.4)	IV.D.A2.2. Analyze evaluation data.
	IV.B.3. Analyze resulting evaluation data.	IV.E.E.1		IV.B.4	IV.D.E.3. Implement appropriate qualitative and quantitative evaluation techniques.				
	IV.B.4. Implement appropriate qualitative and qualitative evaluation techniques.	To Entry IV.D.E.3		NEW	IV.D.E.4. Implement methods to evaluate factors that influence shifts in health status.				
	IV.B.5. Apply evaluation technology as appropriate.	IV.D.A2.1							

Shaded area denotes graduate level competencies

APEND. B

APPEND. B

OLD	Sub-competencies		NEW	Entry (Baccalaureate/Master's, Less Than 5 Years' Experience)		Advanced 1 (Baccalaureate/Master's, 5 Years' Experience or More)		Advanced 2 (Doctorate and 5 Years' Experience or More)	
IV. Competency C: Interpret results of program evaluation. — IV.E	IV.E.A2.1.	IV.C.1. Apply criteria of effectiveness to obtained results of a program.	NEW / IV. Competency E: Interpret results from evaluation and research.	IV.B.3	IV.E.E.1. Analyze evaluation data.	III.D.1	IV.E.A1.1. Compare program activities with the stated program objectives.	IV.C.1	IV.E.A2.1. Determine the achievement of objectives by applying criteria to evaluation results.
	To Advanced IV.E.A2.2	IV.C.2. Translate evaluation results into terms easily understood by others.		NEW	IV.E.E.2. Analyze research data.				
				NEW / IV.C.5	IV.E.E.3. Compare evaluation results to other findings.	IV.C.6	IV.E.A1.2. Develop recommendations based upon evaluation results.	IV.C.2	IV.E.A2.2. Communicate evaluation results using easily understood terms.
	IV.E.E.4	IV.C.3. Report effectiveness of educational programs in achieving proposed objectives.		IV.C.3	IV.E.E.4. Report effectiveness of programs in achieving proposed objectives.				
	LOSS (refer IV.D.A2.2.)	IV.C.4. Implement strategies to analyze data from evaluation assessments.							
	To Entry IV.E.E.3	IV.C.5. Compare evaluation results to other findings.							
	V.E.A1.2	IV.C.6. Make recommendations from evaluation results.							
IV. Competency D: Infer implication from findings for future program planning. — IV.F	To Advanced IV.F.A2.1	IV.D.1. Explore possible explanations for important evaluation findings.	IV.D / IV. Competency F: Infer implications from findings for future health-related activities.			IV.D.2	IV.F.A1.1. Suggest strategies for implementing recommendations that result from evaluation.	Entry IV.D.1	IV.F.A2.1. Propose possible explanations for evaluation findings.
	To Advanced IV.F.A1.1	IV.D.2. Recommend strategies for implementing results of evaluation.							
	LOSS	IV.D.3. Apply findings to refine and maintain programs.				NEW	IV.F.A1.2. Apply evaluation findings to refine and maintain progress.		
	VII.D.A2.2 & IV.F.A1.2.	IV.D.4. Use evaluation findings in policy analysis and development.							
Area of Responsibility V: Coordinating Provision of Health Education Services	**Area of Responsibility V: Coordinating Provision of Health**		**Area of Responsibility V: Administer Health Education Strategies, Interventions, and Programs**						
V. Competency A: Develop a plan for coordinating health education services. — LOSS	I.E.E.1	V.A.1. Determine the extent of available health education services.	NEW / V. Competency A: Exercise organizational leadership.	IX.C.3	V.A.E.1. Conduct strategic planning.	IX.C.4	V.A.A1.1. Develop strategies to reinforce or change organizational culture to achieve program goals.	MAYBE IV.B.1	V.A.A2.1. Facilitate administration of the evaluation plan.
	II.F.E.2	V.A.2. Match health education services to proposed program activities.		NEW / IX.C.1	V.A.E.2. Analyze the organization's culture in relationship to program goals.	NEW	V.A.A1.2. Ensure that program activities comply with existing laws and regulations.		
	I.E.E.2	V.A.3. Identify gaps and overlaps in the provision of collaborative health services.		V.B.I	V.A.E.3. Promote cooperation and feedback among personnel related to the program.	IX.A.2	V.A.A1.3. Develop budgets to support program requirements.		

Shaded area denotes graduate level competencies

OLD		Sub-competencies	NEW	Entry (Baccalaureate/Master's, Less Than 5 Years' Experience)	Advanced 1 (Baccalaureate/Master's, 5 Years' Experience or More)	Advanced 2 (Doctorate and 5 Years' Experience or More)
V. Competency B: Facilitate cooperation between and among levels of program personnel.	LOSS	V.A.E.3 — V.B.1. Promote cooperation and feedback among personnel related to the program.	**V. Competency B: Secure fiscal resources.** NEW		IX.A.2 — V.B.A1.1. Manage program budgets.	IX.A.1 — V.B.A2.1. Prepare proposals to obtain fiscal resources.
		To Advanced V.C.A1.5 — V.B.2. Apply various methods of conflict reduction as needed.				
		VI.D.E.2 — V.B.3. Analyze the role of health educator as liaison between program staff and outside groups and organizations.				
V. Competency C: Formulate practical modes of collaboration among health agencies and organizations.	LOSS	To Advanced V.D.A1.2 — V.C.1. Stimulate development of cooperation among personnel responsible for community health education programs.	**V. Competency C: Manage human resources.** NEW	V.C.E.1. Develop volunteer opportunities. (NEW)	IX.B.4 — V.C.A1.1. Demonstrate leadership in managing human resources.	
					NEW IX.B.5 — V.C.A1.2. Apply human resource policies consistent with relevant laws and regulations.	
		II.B.E.3 — V.C.2. Suggest approaches for integrating health education within existing health programs.			IX.B.1 — V.C.A1.3. Identify qualifications of personnel needed for programs.	
		II.A.E.4 — V.C.3. Develop plans for promoting collaborative efforts among health agencies and organizations with mutual interests.			IX.B.3 — V.C.A1.4. Facilitate staff development.	
		LOSS (refer III.A.E.4) — V.C.4. Organize and facilitate groups, coalitions and partnerships.			V.B.2 — V.C.A1.5. Apply appropriate methods of conflict reduction.	
V. Competency D: Organize in-service training programs for teachers, volunteers, and other interested personnel.	III.D	LOSS — V.D.1. Plan an operational, competency-oriented training program.	**V. Competency D: Obtain acceptance and support for programs.** NEW		IX.D.2 — V.D.A1.1. Use concepts and theories of public relations and communications to obtain program support.	NEW — V.D.A2.1. Provide support for individuals who deliver professional development courses.
		To Advanced III.D.A2.1 — V.D.2. Utilize instructional resources that meet a variety of in-service training needs.				
		To Advanced III.D.A1.1 — V.D.3. Demonstrate a wide range of strategies for conducting in-service training programs.			V.C.1 — V.D.A1.2. Facilitate cooperation among personnel responsible for health education programs.	
		LOSS to VI.D.E.5 — V.D.4. Facilitate collaborative training efforts among health agencies and organizations.				

Shaded area denotes graduate level competencies

APPEND. B

Area of Responsibility VI: OLD — Acting as a Resource Person in Health Education / NEW — Serve as a Health Education Resource Person

OLD Competency	LOSS	Sub-competencies	code	NEW Competency		Entry (Baccalaureate/Master's, Less Than 5 Years' Experience)	code	Advanced 1 (Baccalaureate/Master's, 5 Years' Experience or More)	Advanced 2 (Doctorate and 5 Years' Experience or More)
VI. Competency A: Utilize computerized health information retrieval system effectively.	LOSS	VI.A.1. Match an information need with the appropriate retrieval system.	VI.A.E.I	VI. Competency A: Use health-related information resources.	NEW	VI.A.E.1. Match information needs with the appropriate retrieval systems.	V.I.A.1		
		VI.A.2. Access principal online and other database health information resources.	VI.A.E.4			VI.A.E.2. Select a data system commensurate with program needs.	VI.A.3		
		VI.A.3. Select a data system commensurate with program needs.	To Entry VI.A.E.2			VI.A.E.3. Determine the relevance of various computerized health information resources.	VI.A.4		
		VI.A.4. Determine relevance of various computerized health information resources.	To Entry VI.A.E.3			VI.A.E.4. Access health information resources.	VI.A.2		
		VI.A.5. Assist in establishing and monitoring policies for use of data gathering practices.	LOSS			VI.A.E.5. Employ electronic technology for retrieving references.	NEW (Refer VIII.A.1)		
VI. Competency C: Interpret and respond to requests for health information.	VI.B	VI.C.1. Analyze general processes for identifying the information needed to satisfy a request.	LOSS (refer VI.B.E.1)	VI. Competency B: Respond to requests for health information.	NEW	VI.B.E.1. Identify information sources needed to satisfy a request.	NEW		
		VI.C.2. Employ a wide range of approaches in referring requesters to valid sources of health information.	VI.B.E.2			VI.B.E.2. Refer requesters to valid sources of health information.	VI.C.2		
VI. Competency D: Select effective educational resource materials for dissemination.	VI.C	VI.D.1. Assemble educational material of value to the health of individuals and community groups.	VI.C.E.3	VI. Competency C: Select resource materials for dissemination.	VI.D	VI.C.E.1. Evaluate applicability of resource materials for given audiences.	VI.D.2		
		VI.D.2. Evaluate the worth and applicability of resource materials for given audiences.	VI.C.E.1			VI.C.E.2. Apply various processes to acquire resource materials.	VI.D.3		
		VI.D.3. Apply various processes in the acquisition of resource materials.	VI.C.E.2			VI.C.E.3. Assemble educational material of value to the health of individuals and community groups.	VI.D.1		
		VI.D.4. Compare different methods for distributing educational materials.	VII.B.E.2						
		VI.D.5. Apply communication theory and principles in the development of health education materials.	LOSS						

Shaded area denotes graduate level competencies

OLD	Sub-competencies		NEW		Entry (Baccalaureate/Master's, Less Than 5 Years' Experience)		Advanced 1 (Baccalaureate/Master's, 5 Years' Experience or More)		Advanced 2 (Doctorate and 5 Years' Experience or More)	
VI. Competency B: Establish effective consultative relationships with those requesting assistance in solving health-related problems.	VI.D		VI.B							
	VI.B.1. Analyze parameters of effective consultative relationships.	VI.D.E.1	**VI. Competency D: Establish consultative relationships.**		VI.D.E.1. Analyze parameters of effective consultative relationships.	VI.B.1			VI.D.A2.1. Describe consulting skills needed by health educators.	VI.B.2
	VI.B.2. Describe special skills and abilities needed by health educators for consultation activities.	To Advanced VI.D.A2.1			VI.D.E.2. Analyze the role of the health educator as a liaison between program staff and outside groups and organizations.	V.B.3				
	VI.B.3. Formulate a plan for providing consultation to other health professionals.	LOSS			VI.D.E.3. Act as a liaison among consumer groups, individuals, and health care provider organizations.	VII.D.2				
	VI.B.4. Explain the process of marketing health education consultative services.	LOSS			VI.D.E.4. Apply networking skills to develop and maintain consultative relationships.	VI.B.5				
	VI.B.5. Apply networking skills to develop and maintain consultative relationships.	To Entry VI.D.E.4			VI.D.E.5. Facilitate collaborative training efforts among health agencies and organizations.	V.D.4				

Area of Responsibility VII: Communicating Health and Health Education Needs, Concerns, and Resources (OLD)

Area of Responsibility VII: Communicate and Advocate for Health and Health Education (NEW)

OLD	Sub-competencies		NEW		Entry		Advanced 1		Advanced 2	
VII. Competency A: Interpret concepts, purposes and theories of health education.	LOSS		NEW		NEW					
	VII.A.1. Evaluate the state of the art of health education.	To Advanced VII.C.A2.1	**VII. Competency A: Analyze and respond to current and future needs in health education.**		VII.A.E.1. Analyze factors (e.g., social, cultural, demographic, and political) that influence decision-makers.		VII.A.A1.1. Respond to challenges facing health education programs.	VII.B.5	VII.A.A2.1. Analyze the interrelationships among ethics, values, and behavior.	X.C.1
	VII.A.2. Analyze the foundations of the discipline of health education.	LOSS					VII.A.A1.2. Implement strategies for advocacy initiatives.	NEW	VII.A.A2.2. Relate health education issues to larger social issues.	X.A.1
	VII.A.3. Describe major responsibilities of the health educator in the practice of health education.	To Advanced VII.C.A2.2					VII.A.A1.3. Use evaluation data to advocate for health education programs.	NEW		
	VII.A.4. Articulate the historical and philosophical bases of health education.	LOSS								
VII. Competency C: Select a variety of communication methods and techniques in providing health information.	LOSS		NEW		NEW					
	VII.C.1. Utilize a wide range of techniques for communicating health and health education information.	VII.B.E.5	**VII. Competency B: Apply a variety of communication methods and techniques.**		VII.B.E.1. Assess the appropriateness of language in health education messages.					
	VII.C.2. Demonstrate proficiency in communicating health information and health education needs.	VII.B.E.7			VII.B.E.2. Compare different methods of distributing educational materials.	VI.D.4				

Shaded area denotes graduate level competencies

APEND. B

OLD	Sub-competencies	NEW	Entry (Baccalaureate/Master's, Less Than 5 Years' Experience)	Advanced 1 (Baccalaureate/Master's, 5 Years' Experience or More)	Advanced 2 (Doctorate and 5 Years' Experience or More)
	VII.C.3. Demonstrate both proficiency and accuracy in oral and written presentations.	To Entry VII.B.E.6	VII.B.E.3. Respond to public input regarding health education information. — NEW		
	VII.C.4. Use culturally sensitive communication methods and techniques.	To Entry VII.B.E.4	VII.B.E.4. Use culturally sensitive communication methods and techniques. — VII.C.4		
			VII.B.E.5. Use appropriate techniques when communicating health and health education information. — VII.C.1		
			VII.B.E.6. Use oral, electronic, and written techniques for communicating health education information. — NEW		
			VII.B.E.7. Demonstrate proficiency in communicating health information and health education needs. — VII.C.2		
		VII. Competency C: Promote the health education profession individually and collectively. NEW	VII.C.E.1. Develop a personal plan for professional growth. — X.B.3		VII.C.A2.1. Describe the state-of-the-art of health education practice. — VII.A.1
					VII.C.A2.2. Explain the major responsibilities of the health educator in the practice of health education — VII.A.3
					VII.C.A2.3. Explain the role of health education associations in advancing the profession. — X.B.1
					VII.C.A2.4. Explain the benefits of participating in professional organizations. — NEW (Refer X.B.2)
VII. Competency D: Foster communication between health care providers and consumers. — LOSS	VII.D.1. Interpret the significance and implications of health care providers' messages to consumers.	VII. Competency D: Influence health policy to promote health. NEW	VII.D.E.1. Identify the significance and implications of health care providers' messages to consumers. — VII.D.1	VII.D.A1.1. Use research results to develop health policy. — VIII.C.6	VII.D.A2.1. Describe how research results influence health policy. — VIII.C.5

Shaded area denotes graduate level competencies

OLD	Sub-competencies	NEW	Entry (Baccalaureate/Master's, Less Than 5 Years' Experience)	Advanced 1 (Baccalaureate/Master's, 5 Years' Experience or More)	Advanced 2 (Doctorate and 5 Years' Experience or More)
	VII.D.2. Act as liaison between consumer groups and individuals and health care provider organizations.	VI.D.E.3			VII.D.A2.2. Use evaluation findings in policy analysis and development. IV.D.4
VII. Competency B: Predict the impact of societal value systems on health education programs.	LOSS	I.E.A2.1.			
	VII.B.1. Investigate social forces causing opposing viewpoints regarding health education needs and concerns.				
	VII.B.2. Employ a wide range of strategies for dealing with controversial health issues.	To Advanced III.C.A1.1			
	VII.B.3. Analyze social, cultural, demographic and political factors that influence decision-makers.	To Entry VII.A.E1			
	VII.B.4. Predict future health education needs based upon societal changes.	I.F.A2.1			
	VII.B.5. Respond to challenges to health education programs.	VII.A.A1.1			
Area of Responsibility VIII: Applying Appropriate Research Principles and Methods in Health Education					
VIII. Competency A: Conduct thorough reviews of literature.	VIII.A.1 Employ electronic technology for retrieving references.	To Entry VI.A.E.5			
	VIII.A.2 Analyze references to identify those pertinent to selected health education issues or programs.	To Entry II.D.E.2			
	VIII.A.3 Select and critique sources of health information.	I.A.A2.1			
	VIII.A.4 Evaluate the research design, methodology and findings from the literature.	To Entry IV.A.E.2			
	VIII.A.5 Synthesize key information from the literature.	To Entry IV.A.E.1			
VIII. Competency B: Use appropriate qualitative and quantitative research methods.	VIII.B.1 Assess the merits and limitations of qualitative and quantitative research methods.	IV.A.A2.1			
	VIII.B.2 Apply qualitative and/or quantitative research methods in research designs.	LOSS			

Shaded area denotes graduate level competencies

APEND. B

APEND. B

OLD	Sub-competencies	NEW	Entry *(Baccalaureate/Master's, Less Than 5 Years' Experience)*	Advanced 1 *(Baccalaureate/Master's, 5 Years' Experience or More)*	Advanced 2 *(Doctorate and 5 Years' Experience or More)*
VIII. Competency C: Apply research to health education practice.	VIII.C.1 Use appropriate research methods and designs in assessing needs.	LOSS			
	VIII.C.2 Use information derived from research for program planning.	To Entry II.B.E.1			
	VIII.C.3 Select implementation strategies based upon research results.	II.G.A1.2			
	VIII.C.4 Employ research design, methods and analysis in program evaluation.	LOSS			
	VIII.C.5 Describe how research results inform health policy development.	VII.D.A2.1			
	VIII.C.6 Use research results to inform health policy development.	VII.D.A1.1			
	VIII.C.7 Use protocol for dissemination of research findings.	LOSS			
Area of Responsibility IX: Administering Health Education Programs					
IX Competency A: Develop and manage fiscal resources.	IX.A.1 Prepare proposals to obtain fiscal resources through grants, contract, and other internal and external sources.	V.B.A2.1			
	IX.A.2 Develop and manage realistic budgets to support program requirements.	V.A.A1.3 & V.B.A1.1			
IX. Competency B: Develop and manage human resources.	IX.B.1 Assess and communicate qualifications of personnel needed for programs.	V.C.A1.3			
	IX.B.2 Recruit, employ and evaluate staff members.	LOSS			
	IX.B.3 Provide staff development.	V.C.A1.4			
	IX.B.4 Demonstrate leadership in managing human resources.	V.C.A1.1			

Shaded area denotes graduate level competencies

OLD	Sub-competencies	NEW	Entry (Baccalaureate/Master's, Less Than 5 Years' Experience)	Advanced 1 (Baccalaureate/Master's, 5 Years' Experience or More)	Advanced 2 (Doctorate and 5 Years' Experience or More)
	IX.B.5. Apply human resource policies consistent with relevant laws and regulations.	V.C.A1.2			
IX. Competency C: Exercise organizational leadership.	IX.C.1 Analyze the organization's culture in relationship to program goals.	To Entry V.A.E.2			
	IX.C.2 Assess the political climate of the organization, community, state and nation regarding conditions that advance or inhibit the goals of the program.	I.E.A1.1.			
	IX.C.3 Conduct long-range and strategic planning.	To Entry V.A.E.1			
	IX.C.4 Develop strategies to reinforce or change organizational culture to achieve program goals.	V.A.A1.1.			
	IX.C.5 Develop strategies to influence public policy.	LOSS			
IX. Competency D: Obtain acceptance and support for programs.	IX.D.1 Apply social marketing principles and techniques to achieve program goals.	LOSS			
	IX.D.2 Employ concepts and theories of public relations and communications to obtain program support.	V.D.A1.1			
	IX.D.3 Incorporate demographically and culturally sensitive techniques to promote programs.	To Entry III.C.E.4			
	IX.D.4 Use needs assessment information to advocate for health education programs.	LOSS			
Area of Responsibility X: Advancing the Profession of Health Education					
X. Competency A: Provide a critical analysis of current and future needs in	X.A.1 Relate health education issues to larger social issues.	VII.A.A2.2			

Shaded area denotes graduate level competencies

APEND. B

OLD	Sub-competencies	NEW	Entry (Baccalaureate/Master's, Less Than 5 Years' Experience)		Advanced 1 (Baccalaureate/Master's, 5 Years' Experience or More)		Advanced 2 (Doctorate and 5 Years' Experience or More)	
health education.	X.A.2 Articulate health education's role in policy formation at various organizational and community levels. LOSS							
X. Competency B: Assume responsibility for advancing the profession.	X.B.1 Analyze the role of the health education associations in advancing the profession. VII.C.A2.3							
	X.B.2 Participate in professional organization. LOSS (refer VII.C.A2.4)							
	X.B.3 Develop a personal plan for professional growth. To Entry VII.C.E.1							
X. Competency C: Apply ethical principles as they relate to the practice of health education.	X.C.1 Analyze the interrelationships among ethics, values and behavior. VII.A.A1.1							
	X.C.2 Relate the importance of a code of ethics to professional practice. LOSS (refer III.CE.1)							
	X.C.3 Subscribe to a professionally recognized health education code of ethics. To Entry III.C.E.1							

Shaded area denotes graduate level competencies

Detailed Summary of Changes

Area of Responsibility I
Competency A: Unchanged
Sub-competencies: Two new (I.A.E.1; I.A.E.4.) at entry level
Two unchanged at entry level
One unchanged at Advanced level 2

Competency B: Unchanged
Sub-competencies: One new at entry level (I.B.E.4)
Two unchanged at entry level
One unchanged (old graduate) at entry level (old I.A.5)
None present at advanced levels

Competency C: Content unchanged, but is the old I.B
Sub-competencies: None new at entry level
Two unchanged at entry level
One unchanged at Advanced level 1

Competency D: New
Sub-competencies: None listed at entry level
Two new at Advanced level 1
One new at Advanced level 2

Competency E: New
Sub-competencies: Two unchanged at entry level
One unchanged at Advanced level 1
One unchanged at Advanced level 2

Competency F: Unchanged
Sub-competencies: One unchanged at entry level
One unchanged at Advanced level 1
One unchanged at Advanced level 2

Area of Responsibility II
Competency A: Essentially unchanged
Sub-competencies: One new at entry level
Three unchanged at entry level
One unchanged at Advanced level 1

Competency B: New
Sub-competencies: Two unchanged at entry level
Two unchanged (old graduate) at entry level
(VIII.C.2; II.A.5)
One new at Advanced level 1

Competency C: Essentially unchanged
Sub-competencies: One new at entry level
Three new at Advanced level 1
One unchanged at Advanced level 1
Two unchanged at Advanced level 2

Competency D: Essentially unchanged
Sub-competencies: Two unchanged at entry level
Two unchanged at Advanced level 1
One unchanged at Advanced level 2

Competency E: Essentially unchanged
Sub-competencies: None listed at entry level
Two unchanged at Advanced level 1
Three unchanged at Advanced level 2

Competency F: Unchanged
Sub-competencies: One unchanged at entry level
One new (old graduate) at entry level (III.C.4)
Two new at Advanced level 1
One new at Advanced level 2

Competency G: New
Sub-competencies: One new at entry level
One unchanged at entry level
Two unchanged at Advanced level 1

Area of Responsibility III
Competency A: New
Sub-competencies: One new at entry level
Two similar to old graduate competencies at entry level
One unchanged at entry level
One unchanged at Advanced level 1

Competency B: New
Sub-competencies: One unchanged at entry level
One new at entry level
One unchanged at Advanced level 1
One new at Advanced level 1
One unchanged at Advanced level 2

Competency C: New
Sub-competencies: Two new at entry level
Three unchanged (old graduate) at entry level (X.C.3; III.C.5; IX.D.3)
One unchanged at Advanced level 1

Competency D: Essentially unchanged
Sub-competencies: None listed at entry level
One unchanged at Advanced level 1
One unchanged at Advanced level 2

Area of Responsibility IV
Competency A: New
Sub-competencies: Two unchanged (old graduate) at entry level (VIII.A.5; VIII.A.4)
One unchanged at Advanced level 1
One unchanged at Advanced level 2

Competency B: New
Sub-competencies: One unchanged (old graduate) at entry level (IV.A.6)
One new at entry level
Two unchanged at Advanced level 1
One new at Advanced level 1
Two unchanged at Advanced level 2

Competency C: New
Sub-competencies: One new at entry level
One unchanged (old graduate) at entry level (IV.A.8)

Competency D: New
Sub-competencies: Two new at entry level
One unchanged at entry level
One unchanged (old graduate) at entry level (IV.B.4)
One unchanged at Advanced level 1
One unchanged at Advanced level 2
One new at Advanced level 2

Competency E: New
Sub-competencies: Two unchanged at entry level
One unchanged (old graduate) at entry level (IV.C.5)
One new at entry level
Two unchanged at Advanced level 1
Two unchanged at Advanced level 2

Competency F: Unchanged
Sub-competencies: None listed at entry level
One new at Advanced level 1
One unchanged at Advanced level 1
One unchanged at Advanced level 2

Area of Responsibility V
Competency A: New
Sub-competencies: One unchanged at entry level
Two new (old graduate) at entry level (IX.C.3; IX.C.1)
Two unchanged at Advanced level 1
One new at Advanced level 1
One unchanged at Advanced level 2

Competency B: New
Sub-competencies: None listed at entry level
One unchanged at Advanced level 1
One unchanged at Advanced level 2

Competency C: New
Sub-competencies: One new at entry level
One new (old graduate) at entry level (IX.B.5)
Three unchanged at Advanced level 1

Competency D: New
Sub-competencies: None listed at entry level
Two unchanged at Advanced level 1
One new at Advanced level 2

Area of Responsibility VI
Competency A: New
Sub-competencies: Two unchanged at entry level
Three unchanged (old graduate) at entry level
(VI.A.3; VI.A.4; VIII.A.1)

Competency B: Unchanged
Sub-competencies: One new at entry level
One unchanged at entry level

Competency C: Unchanged
Sub-competencies: Three unchanged at entry level

Competency D: Unchanged
Sub-competencies: Three unchanged at entry level
Two unchanged (old graduate) at entry level
(VI.B.5; V.D.4)
One unchanged at Advanced level 2

Area of Responsibility VII
Competency A: New
Sub-competencies: One unchanged (old graduate) at entry level (VII.B.3)
One unchanged at Advanced level 1
Two new at Advanced level 1
Two unchanged at Advanced level 2

Competency B: New
Sub-competencies: Three new at entry level
Three unchanged at entry level
One unchanged (old graduate) at entry level (VII.C.4)

Competency C: New
Sub-competencies: One new (old graduate) at entry level (X.B.3)
Three unchanged at Advanced level 2
One new at Advanced level 2

Competency D: New
Sub-competencies: One unchanged at entry level
One unchanged at Advanced level 1
Two unchanged at Advanced level 2

Committees of the Competencies Update Project and Earlier Competency-Related Works

In addition to the various committees of the Competencies Update Project itself, this appendix lists those individuals who served on previous committees defining the role and competencies of the health educator.

National Health Educator Competencies Update Project Advisory Committee (1998-2004)

Steering Committee:
Dr. Gary Gilmore, CUP Chair
Dr. Larry Olsen
Dr. Alyson Taub

Members:
Ms. Elaine Auld
Dr. David R. Black
Dr. Tom Butler
Dr. Ellen M. Capwell
Dr. Helen Welle Graf
Ms. Barbara Hager
Ms. Linda Lysoby
Dr. Beverly Mahoney
Dr. Mary Marks
Dr. Marion Micke
Dr. Kathleen Miner
Dr. Sheila M. Patterson
Dr. Susan Radius
Dr. Edmund Ricci
Dr. John Sciacca
Dr. Becky Smith
Dr. Margaret Smith
Dr. Carol Soha
Ms. Lori Stegmier
Dr. Stephen H. Stewart
Ms. Emily Tyler

CUP Data Analysis Group (2003-2004)

Dr. Randy Black
Dr. Dave Connell
Dr. Dan Coster
Dr. Gary Gilmore

Dr. Kathy Miner
Dr. Larry Olsen
Dr. Alyson Taub

Joint Committee for the Development of Graduate-Level Preparation Standards (1992-1996)

Co-Chairpersons:
Dr. Margaret M. Smith
Dr. Stephen H. Stewart

Members:
Dr. Evelyn E. Ames
Dr. Donald L. Calitri
Dr. William B. Cissell
Ms. Patricia P. Evans
Ms. Mary E. Hawkins
Mr. Douglas Rippler
Dr. Mark J. Kittleson
Dr. William C. Livingood, Jr.
Capt. Patricia D. Mail
Dr. Carl J. Peter
Dr. Donald A. Read
Ms. Ruth Richards
Dr. James Robinson III
Dr. Elaine M. Vitello

Graduate Competencies Writing Ad Hoc Committee (1997)

Ms. Patricia P. Evans
Dr. William C. Livingood, Jr.
Capt. Patricia D. Mail
Dr. James Robinson
Dr. Margaret M. Smith
Dr. Alyson Taub

Graduate Competencies Implementation Committee (1997-1998)

Ms. Elaine Auld
Dr. Ellen M. Capwell
Dr. William B. Cissell

Mr. William B. Cosgrove
Ms. Patricia P. Evans
Ms. Aileen Frazee
Dr. Gary D. Gilmore
Dr. Audrey Gotsch
Dr. William C. Livingood, Jr.
Dr. Sheila M. Patterson
Dr. James Robinson
Dr. Louis Rowitz
Dr. Becky J. Smith
Dr. Margaret M. Smith
Dr. Stephen H. Stewart
Dr. Alyson Taub
Dr. Elaine M. Vitello

**National Task Force on the Preparation and Practice
of Health Educators (1978-1988)**

Dr. John Burt*
Dr. Helen Cleary, Chair, Founder*
Dr. Peter Cortese, Vice Chair, Co-founder*
Dr. William Carlyon*
Dr. William B. Cissell
Dr. John Cooper
Dr. Bryan Cooke
Dr. Robert H. Conn*
Dr. Wanda H. Judd
Ms. Elizabeth Lee
Rev. Robert McEwen
Dr. Mabel Robinson*
Dr. Helen S. Ross*
Ms. Helen Savage
Dr. Warren Schaller*
Dr. Becky J. Smith
Mr. Leonard Tritsch
Dr. Alyson Taub
Dr. Elaine M. Vitello
Dr. Joan M. Wolle*
Ms. Anna Skiff, MPH, Volunteer Staff

*Original Task Force Members

Competency Matrices

Directions for Use of the Area Matrices

For each level of practice, a matrix is provided for each of the seven areas of respon sibility. In the indicated column, enter the course number and title of each professional preparation course required of health education majors enrolled in your program. Remember that for each level of practice all competencies and sub-competencies of the previous level(s) must also be mastered. Each course listed should be rated only by faculty currently responsible for its instruction, whether the course is taught by faculty within or outside the department.

Referring to the competencies and sub-competencies, the instructor is to indicate whether or not each of the sub-competencies is currently being taught as an integral part of the course. Remember that a competency statement is not just some amount of subject matter preceded by a behavioral skill. The statement must be viewed as a whole. The question each instructor must answer in connection with every competency and sub-competency specified in the area matrices is "Are the students taking this course learning to perform the described competency, or are they merely learning asso-ciated subject matter?" Obviously, the instructor of each course is more qualified than any other faculty member to make that judgment.

If a sub-competency is given major emphasis and practice as part of a course, the instructor places the number 2 in the corresponding box. If the sub-competency receives at least minor study and practice in the course, the number 1 is assigned. In the event that a sub-competency is not a part of the study of that course, a zero is assigned. Figure 1 illustrates such an analysis of four exemplary health education courses. As each matrix is completed, total the recorded data to answer the following questions: (1) Of the possible number of sub-competencies listed for the area of responsibility, how many are being addressed to some degree? (2) Are there any sub-competencies or competencies not touched upon by any course in the program? (3) Which of the cours-es contribute the most to achievement of the competencies identified as essential in carrying out the area of responsibility?

Directions for Use of the Analysis Matrix

When all of the area matrices have been completed, the eighth matrix, the horizontal analysis matrix, is used as an organizing and summarizing tool. The horizontal analysis matrix is designed to facilitate organization of the combined data obtained by means of the seven area matrices. The same courses that appeared on the area matrices are listed along the vertical axis. The data recorded on the seven area matrices should be transferred by the department chair or designate.

Notice that for each area of responsibility, the competencies are indicated by letters (A, B, C, etc.) across the horizontal axis. Below each letter the total number of support-ive sub-competencies is indicated in parentheses as 4, 3, 2, and so on.

In each completed area matrix, and for every course listed, enter the number of sub-competencies given a rating of 2 and the number of those given a rating of 1 in the appropriate box (see Figure 2).

APEND. D

As an example, suppose that of four sub-competencies specified as essential to the achievement of Competency A, area of responsibility I, at the entry level, the instructor of a course has reported that two sub-competencies receive major emphasis and the other two are given at least some emphasis. The number given major emphasis (in this case 2) is entered in the top portion of the box, and the number given minor emphasis (which is also 2) is entered in the lower portion, so that it looks like a fraction (2/2). As another example, for Competency B, which has four sub-competencies, none are reported as being given major emphasis, but four are receiving some emphasis. These data would be recorded as 0 (zeros) and need not be indicated or counted as they contribute nothing to the total scores.

When all of the data have been entered for all of the courses and for all seven areas of responsibility, total and enter in the column at the right the number of sub-competencies reported as receiving major and minor emphasis with reference to each course. Next, total each column vertically. The resulting figure represents the coverage of that competency as the outcome of the entire program. In adding these columns, include both figures of the "fraction," so that 2/2 adds 4 to the total, whereas 2/0 would add only 2 to the total.

Consider Competency A, area of responsibility I, once again. Because there are four sub-competencies, complete coverage of that competency within a single course would be represented by the number 4. To assess the emphasis given to that competency as the outcome of the entire program of studies, add the reported numbers in the appropriate column. When given ten courses, the greatest possible coverage of Competency A would be indicated by a score of 40.

It is highly unlikely that any one course will encompass consideration of all of the sub-competencies or even all of the areas of responsibility. However, taken together, what should emerge from the matrix survey is a graphic analysis of an existing curriculum through the 29 competencies and the 82 sub-competencies at the Entry level, the 26 competencies and 48 sub-competencies at Advanced 1 level, and the 22 competencies and 33 sub-competencies at the Advanced 2 level, as well as information regarding the depth to which each of them is being studied. Again, it must be stressed that all previous competencies must be mastered in addition to the competencies at the current level. The balance, or lack of it, in time and emphasis accorded each of the areas of responsibility should also be apparent.

Purpose of the Matrix Surveys

The purpose of the matrix surveys is to provide data concerning the current degree of relevance between existing course content and that implicit in the defined competencies; to identify strengths and weaknesses of a curriculum with regard to information; and to establish a starting point for any subsequent program revisions, adaptations, or additions that are decided upon.

The completed horizontal analysis matrix answers most of the basic questions that curriculum decision-makers might ask about an existing program of courses in light of its potential adaptability to the competency-based plan. If more specific information is needed, the appropriate area matrix will provide some answers. In other words, the horizontal matrix might show that three out of four sub-competencies for Competency B, area of responsibility 1, are given only minor consideration and the other one is not covered at all. The area matrix indicates which sub-competency is omitted and which are given slight coverage.

Together, the matrices afford curriculum decision-makers quick answers to questions such as the following:

1. How many of the competencies are currently being addressed by the curriculum?
2. How many of the sub-competencies receive major emphasis in the program, as shown by a rating of 2?
3. How many of the sub-competencies receive at least minor study, as shown by a rating of 1?
4. If there are competencies not now receiving any attention at all, which are they, and in what area(s) are they found?
5. In each of the areas of responsibility, how many sub-competencies are not being addressed?
6. Which courses are providing broadest coverage and which are providing least coverage of the seven areas of responsibility?
7. Are there any areas of responsibility that now receive little if any consideration in the curriculum? If so, which ones?
8. Are there courses that appear to be irrelevant to the competencies, as reflected in the number of zeros shown? If so, could this be changed without giving up the course itself?
9. What implications do you see in these data for course revision, course modification, or the development of new courses?

It is probable that the data obtained about a traditional professional preparation program in health education will show that it is not so much the content of existing courses that would have to be changed in adopting a competency-based plan. Rather, it would be a new perspective on course goals and objectives, as well as an increased use of experiential teaching-learning methods to address all areas of the competency-based model. In any case, practice of all of the competencies for each area of responsibility should be included in some instructional activity in a logically appropriate course.

Adapting Existing Curricula

Once the faculty has analyzed each of the courses currently offered and required of prospective health educators, it should be clear what changes will be needed. Each faculty member should be charged with making the revisions necessary to better the fit between his or her course objectives and achievement of the competencies. All of the faculty should participate in planning and designing any new courses deemed necessary to facilitate implementation of competencies now being completely overlooked.

Developing New Curricula

All of this discussion has looked at the problem of implementing a competency-based curriculum from the perspective of an already existing program. Where there is

APEND. D

no program in existence, a matrix survey would not be possible. Individuals charged with developing a brand new curriculum would start with the professional preparation curricula recommended by health education authorities, and professional groups would suggest an accepted starting point of courses to which the competencies could logically be assigned.

In arriving at decisions about where a competency is to be taught, it is advisable to take an experimental approach. That is, decisions reached at this point need to be regarded as tentative and subject to change through trial and evaluation by students, faculty, and employers of the program's graduates. Several years of evaluation and modification may be necessary before there is assurance that the curriculum plan is providing all of the learning potential possible. Moreover, it should be remembered that the competency framework presented here is also in the process of evolution. If it were otherwise, then health education would cease to grow and develop as a discipline and as a profession.

Selecting Teaching-Learning Strategies

It is not the function of a curriculum framework to specify or describe learning opportunities or lesson plans. Criteria for the selection of a teaching strategy include the following: (1) it must provide practice in the skill specified in the objective; (2) it must arrange for the discovery or introduction of the content; (3) the activities must be satisfying to the learner; (4) the activities must be appropriate to the past experience and present abilities of the learner; and (5) if several strategies meet the preceding criteria, the one chosen should be the strategy most likely to produce more than one positive outcome.

In general, experiential learning is more effective than passive learning in promoting competency. Everyone learns better by doing than by watching or listening. All in all, the best teaching-learning strategy is the one that encourages learners to practice doing what the objective proposes that they need to learn to do.

The Competency Framework by Areas of Responsibility

Each of the seven areas of responsibility constituting the competency-based curriculum framework is introduced by a discussion of the area itself in Section III. A general statement is provided that describes the area of responsibility in broad terms: its purpose, its meaning, the form it takes in health education, and its relation to the other areas.

The competency framework for each area is developed hierarchically as a set of competency statements, each of which is supported by more specific and narrowly drawn sub-competencies, upon which in turn measurable general objectives are based and proposed. The sequence in which the areas of responsibility are presented is more or less logical, not absolute. No priorities are intended, nor should any be presumed.

FIGURE 1

Area of Responsibility I Matrix
Assess Individual and Community Needs for Health Education

Entry

Course Title	Comp A Subcomp				Comp B Subcomp				Comp C Subcomp		Comp E Subcomp		Comp F Subcomp	Total by Course Max = 13
	1	2	3	4	1	2	3	4	1	2	1	2	1	
Community Health	2	2	1	1	1	1	1	1	1	2	1	2	1	12
Biostatistics	0	0	0	0	0	0	0	0	2	2	1	0	2	2
Administration	1	0	0	0	2	2	1	1	0	0	0	0	1	10
School Health	2	2	1	2	2	1	1	0	2	2	2	2	1	12
Etc.														

Total by Area
Maximum = 13 times
Number of courses

Advanced I

Course Title	Comp C Subcomp	Comp D Subcomp		Comp E Subcomp	Comp F Subcomp
	1	1	2	1	1

Advanced II

Course Title	Comp A Subcomp	Comp D Subcomp	Comp E Subcomp	Comp F Subcomp	Total by Course Max = 9
	1	1	1	1	

Total by Area
Maximum = 22 times
Number of courses

Code: 2 = Major emphasis: 1 = Minor emphasis: 0 = emphasis

APEND. D

FIGURE 2

Entry- Level
Analysis Sheet: Areas of Responsibility

Competencies / Sub-competencies

Course Title	Area I A (4)	Area I B (2)	Area I C (2)	Area I E (2)	Area I F (1)	Area II A (4)	Area II B (4)	Area II C (4)	Area II D (1)	Area II F (2)	Area II G (2)	Area III A (4)	Area III B (2)	Area III C (5)	Area IV A (2)	Area IV B (2)	Area IV C (2)	Area IV D (4)	Area IV E (4)	Area V A (3)	Area V C (1)	Area VI A (5)	Area VI B (2)	Area VI C (3)	Area VI D (5)	Area VII A (1)	Area VII B (7)	Area VII C (1)	Area VII D (1)	Total Comp By Course
Community Health	2 / 2	0 / 4	2 / 0	0 / 1	0 / 1																									
Biostatistics	0 / 0	0 / 0	0 / 1	0 / 0	1 / 0																									
Administration	0 / 1	2 / 2	0 / 0	0 / 0	0 / 1																									
School Health	3 / 1	2 / 1	2 / 0	2 / 0	0 / 1																									
Etc.																														
SubTotal	9	11	5	3	4																									
Proposed New Courses																														

Subtotal = Possible coverage of each competency based upon the number of sub-competencies times the number of course titles (for example, given 10 courses, the greatest coverage possible of Area I, Competency A, would be 40).

APEND. D

Area of Responsibility I Matrix
Assess Individual and Community Needs for Health Education

Entry

Course Title	Comp A Subcomp 1	2	3	4	Comp B Subcomp 1	2	3	4	Comp C Subcomp 1	2	Comp E Subcomp 1	2	Comp F Subcomp 1	Total by Course Max = 13

Total by Area
Maximum = 13 times
Number of courses

Advanced I

Course Title	Comp C Subcomp 1	Comp D Subcomp 1	2	Comp E Subcomp 1	Comp F Subcomp 1

Advanced II

Course Title	Comp A Subcomp 1	Comp D Subcomp 1	Comp E Subcomp 1	Comp F Subcomp 1	Total by Course Max = 9

Total by Area
Maximum = 22 times
Number of courses

Code: 2 = Major emphasis: 1 = Minor emphasis: 0 = emphasis

APEND. D

Area of Responsibility II Matrix
Plan Health Education Strategies, Interventions, and Programs

Entry

Course Title	Comp A Subcomp 1 2 3 4	Comp B Subcomp 1 2 3 4	Comp C Subcomp 1	Comp D Subcomp 1 2	Comp F Subcomp 1 2	Comp G Subcomp 1 2	Total by Course Max = 15

Total by Area
Maximum = 15 times
Number of courses

Advanced I

Course Title	Comp A Subcomp 1	Comp B Subcomp 1	Comp C Subcomp 1 2 3 4	Comp D Subcomp 1	Comp E Subcomp 1 2	Comp F Subcomp 1 2	Comp G Subcomp 1 2	Comp C Subcomp 1 2	Comp D Subcomp 1	Comp E Subcomp 1 2 3	Comp F Subcomp 1	Total by Course Max = 21

Advanced II

Total by Area
Maximum = 36 times
Number of courses

Code: 2 = Major emphasis: 1 = Minor emphasis: 0 = emphasis

APEND. D

Area of Responsibility III Matrix

Implement Health Education Strategies, Interventions, and Programs

Entry

Course Title	Comp A Subcomp				Comp B Subcomp		Comp C Subcomp					Total by Course Max = 11
	1	2	3	4	1	2	1	2	3	4	5	

Total by Area
Maximum = 11 times
Number of courses

Advanced I

Course Title	Comp A Subcomp	Comp B Subcomp		Comp C Subcomp	Comp D Subcomp	
	1	1	2	1	1	

Advanced II

	Comp B Subcomp	Comp D Subcomp	Total by Course Max = 7
	1	1	

Total by Area
Maximum = 18 times
Number of courses

Code: 2 = Major emphasis: 1 = Minor emphasis: 0 = emphasis

APEND. D

Area of Responsibility IV Matrix
Conduct Evaluation and Research Related to Health Education

Entry

Course Title	Comp A Subcomp 1	Comp A Subcomp 2	Comp B Subcomp 1	Comp B Subcomp 2	Comp C Subcomp 1	Comp C Subcomp 2	Comp D Subcomp 1	Comp D Subcomp 2	Comp D Subcomp 3	Comp D Subcomp 4	Comp E Subcomp 1	Comp E Subcomp 2	Comp E Subcomp 3	Comp E Subcomp 4	Total by Course Max = 14

Total by Area
Maximum = 14 times
Number of courses

Advanced I

Course Title	Comp A Subcomp 1	Comp B Subcomp 1	Comp B Subcomp 2	Comp B Subcomp 3	Comp D Subcomp 1	Comp E Subcomp 1	Comp E Subcomp 2	Comp F Subcomp 1	Comp F Subcomp 2

Advanced II

	Comp A Subcomp 1	Comp B Subcomp 1	Comp B Subcomp 2	Comp D Subcomp 1	Comp D Subcomp 2	Comp E Subcomp 1	Comp E Subcomp 2	Comp F Subcomp 1	Total by Course Max = 17

Total by Area
Maximum = 31 times
Number of courses

Code: 2 = Major emphasis: 1 = Minor emphasis: 0 = emphasis

Area of Responsibility V Matrix

Administer Health Education Strategies, Interventions, and Programs

Course Title	Comp A Subcomp			Comp C Subcomp	Total by Course Max = 4
	1	2	3	1	

Total by Area
Maximum = 4 times
Number of courses

Advanced I

Course Title	Comp A Subcomp			Comp B Subcomp	Comp C Subcomp					Comp D Subcomp
	1	2	3	1	1	2	3	4	5	1

Advanced II

Comp A Subcomp	Comp B Subcomp	Comp D Subcomp	Total by Course Max = 14
1	1	1	

Total by Area
Maximum = 18 times
Number of courses

Code: 2 = Major emphasis: 1 = Minor emphasis: 0 = emphasis

Area of Responsibility VI Matrix
Serve as a Health Education Resource Person

Entry

Course Title	Comp A Subcomp					Comp B Subcomp		Comp C Subcomp			Comp D Subcomp					Total by Course Max = 15
	1	2	3	4	5	1	2	1	2	3	1	2	3	4	5	

Total by Area
Maximum = 15 times
Number of courses

Advanced II

Course Title	Comp D Subcomp 1	Total by Course Max = 1

Total by Area
Maximum = 16 times
Number of courses

Code: 2 = Major emphasis: 1 = Minor emphasis: 0 = emphasis

APEND. D

APEND. D

Area of Responsibility VII Matrix
Communicate and Advocate for Health and Health Education

Entry

Course Title	Comp A Subcomp 1	Comp B Subcomp 1	Comp B Subcomp 2	Comp B Subcomp 3	Comp B Subcomp 4	Comp B Subcomp 5	Comp B Subcomp 6	Comp B Subcomp 7	Comp C Subcomp 1	Comp D Subcomp 1	Total by Course Max = 10

Total by Area
Maximum = 10 times
Number of courses

Advanced I

Course Title	Comp A Subcomp 1	Comp A Subcomp 2	Comp A Subcomp 3	Comp D Subcomp 1

Advanced II

Course Title	Comp A Subcomp 1	Comp A Subcomp 2	Comp C Subcomp 1	Comp C Subcomp 2	Comp C Subcomp 3	Comp C Subcomp 4	Comp D Subcomp 1	Comp D Subcomp 2	Total by Course Max = 12

Total by Area
Maximum = 22 times
Number of courses

Code: 2 = Major emphasis: 1 = Minor emphasis: 0 = emphasis

Entry- Level
Analysis Sheet: Areas of Responsibility

Competencies
Sub-competencies

Course Title	Area I					Area II						Area III			Area IV					Area V		Area VI				Area VII				Total Comp By Course
	A	B	C	E	F	A	B	C	D	F	G	A	B	C	A	B	C	D	E	A	C	A	B	C	D	A	B	C	D	
	4	2	2	1	4	4	1	2	2	4	2	5	2	2	2	2	4	4	3	1	5	2	3	5	1	7	1	1	1	
SubTotal																														
Proposed New Courses																														

Subtotal = Possible coverage of each competency based upon the number of sub-competencies times the number of course titles (for example, given 10 courses, the greatest coverage possible of Area I, Competency A, would be 40).

APEND. D

Advanced I
Analysis Sheet: Areas of Responsibility

Competencies

Course Title	Area I				Area II							Area III				Area IV					Area V				Area VII		Total Comp by Course
	C	D	E	F	A	B	C	D	E	F	G	A	B	C	D	A	B	D	E	F	A	B	C	D	A	D	

Sub-competencies

	1	2	1	1	1	1	1	4	2	2	2	2	1	1	1	3	1	2	2	3	1	5	2	3	1		
SubTotal																											
Proposed New Courses																											

Subtotal = Possible coverage of each competency based upon the number of sub-competencies times the number of course titles (for example, given 10 courses, the greatest coverage possible of Area I, Competency A, would be 40).

APEND. D

Advanced II
Analysis Sheet: Areas of Responsibility

Course Title	Area I				Area II				Area III		Area IV					Area V			Area VI	Area VII			Total Comp by Course
Competencies	A	D	E	F	C	D	E	F	B	D	A	B	D	E	F	A	B	D	D	A	C	D	
Sub-competencies	1	1	1	1	2	1	3	1	1	1	1	2	2	2	1	1	1	1	1	2	4	2	
SubTotal																							
Proposed New Courses																							

Subtotal = Possible coverage of each competency based upon the number of sub-competencies times the number of course titles (for example, given 10 courses, the greatest coverage possible of Area I, Competency A, would be 40).

Notes

A Competency-Based Framework for Health Educators – 2006